Otolaryngology

SPECIALTY BOARD REVIEW

Otolaryngology

630
Questions & Answers

J. Michael Willett, MDCM, FRCS(C)
Clinical Lecturer
Department of Otolaryngology
Yale University School of Medicine
Co-Director, Facial Plastic Surgery
Southern New England Ear, Nose, Throat and Facial Plastic Surgery Group
President, New England Facial Plastic Surgery Society
Attending Otolaryngologist
Hospital of Saint Raphael
Attending Otolaryngologist
Yale-New Haven Hospital
New Haven, Connecticut

K.J. Lee, MD, FACS
Associate Clinical Professor
Department of Otolaryngology
Yale University School of Medicine
Director, Ear Research and Education Center
Director, Laser Surgery Center
Director, Southern New England Ear, Nose, Throat
and Facial Plastic Surgery Group
Chief of Otolaryngology
Hospital of Saint Raphael
Attending Otolaryngologist
Yale-New Haven Hospital
New Haven, Connecticut

APPLETON & LANGE
Norwalk, Connecticut

Notice: The authors and the publisher of this volume have taken care to make certain that the doses of drugs and schedules of treatment are correct and compatible with the standards generally accepted at the time of publication. Nevertheless, as new information becomes available, changes in treatment and in the use of drugs become necessary. The reader is advised to carefully consult the instruction and information material included in the package insert of each drug or therapeutic agent before administration. This advice is especially important when using new or infrequently used drugs. The publisher disclaims any liability, loss, injury, or damage incurred as a consequence, directly or indirectly, or the use and application of any of the contents of the volume.

Prentice Hall International (UK) Limited, *London*
Prentice Hall of Australia Pty. Limited, *Sydney*
Prentice Hall Canada, Inc., *Toronto*
Prentice Hall Hispanoamericana, S.A., *Mexico*
Prentice Hall of India Private Limited, *New Delhi*
Prentice Hall of Japan, Inc., *Tokyo*
Simon & Schuster Asia Pte. Ltd., *Singapore*
Editora Prentice Hall do Brasil Ltda., *Rio de Janeiro*
Prentice Hall, *Englewood Cliffs, New Jersey*

ISBN: 0-8385-7580-3
ISSN: 1077-2057

Acquisitions Editor: J. Alex Schwartz
Production Editor: Jennifer Sinsavich
Cover Designer: Libby Schmitz

ISBN 0-8385-7580-3

I wish to thank my wife, Evelyn, and children, Sarah, Jordan, and Jessica for their love and understanding. I also would like to thank my co-editor, Dr. K.J. Lee, for his support and leadership in the formulation of this text. A special thank you is extended to Evelyn, who helped with the preparation of questions and transcription of the text.

JMW

Contents

Preface xi

Introduction xiii

1. Anatomy of the Ear 1
   Answers and Discussion...5

2. Audiology...8
   Answers and Discussion..16

3. Electrical Response Audiometry....................................19
   Answers and Discussion..22

4. The Vestibular System and Its Disorders, Part I.........24
   Answers and Discussion..27

5. The Vestibular System and Its Disorders, Part II........29
   Answers and Discussion..32

6. Speech, Language, and Voice 34
   Answers and Discussion..37

7. Congenital Deafness..39
   Answers and Discussion..46

8. Cochlear Implants 51
   Answers and Discussion...54

9. Neurotology and Skull Base Surgery 56
   Answers and Discussion...59

10. Facial Nerve Paralysis..61
    Answers and Discussion...66

11. Syndromes and Eponyms..69
    Answers and Discussion...73

12. Embryology of Clefts and Pouches.............................76
    Answers and Discussion...79

13. Cleft Lip and Palate..81
    Answers and Discussion...85

14. Immunology and Allergy 88
    Answers and Discussion...91

15. The Chest...93
    Answers and Discussion...100

16. Related Ophthalmology..103
    Answers and Discussion...106

17. Related Neurology...108
    Answers and Discussion...112

18. Fluids, Electrolytes, and Acid–Base Balance...............114
    Answers and Discussion...117

19. Surgical Hemostasis 119
    Answers and Discussion...124

20. Cancer Chemotherapy 127
    Answers and Discussion...130

21. Nasal Endoscopy and Its Surgical Applications 132
    Answers and Discussion...136

22. Antimicrobial Therapy in Head and Neck Surgery...................138
    Answers and Discussion...142

23. Nutritional Assessment and Support...........................144
    Answers and Discussion...147

24. Neck Spaces and Facial Planes 149
    Answers and Discussion...151

25. The Oral Cavity, Oropharynx, and Hypopharynx.....................153
    Answers and Discussion...158

26. The Esophagus 161
    Answers and Discussion...165

27. Swallowing Disorders 168
    Answers and Discussion...171

28. The Salivary Glands: Benign and Malignant Disease...............173
    Answers and Discussion...178

29. Carcinoma of the Oral Cavity and Pharynx 182
    Answers and Discussion...186

30. Cancer of the Larynx, Ear, and Paranasal Sinus 189
    Answers and Discussion...193

31. Thyroid and Parathyroid Glands 195
    Answers and Discussion...198

32. Carotid Body Tumor, Hemangioma, Lymphangioma,
    Melanoma, Cysts, and Tumors of the Jaw 200
    Answers and Discussion...203

33. Infections of the Ear 205
    Answers and Discussion...209

34. Noninfectious Diseases of the Ear 212
    Answers and Discussion...217

x / Contents

35. The Nose and Sinuses 219
     Answers and Discussion..224

36. The Larynx 227
     Answers and Discussion..231

37. Sleep Apnea..234
     Answers and Discussion..238

38. Facial and Airway Trauma......................................240
     Answers and Discussion..244

39. Pediatric Otolaryngology 247
     Answers and Discussion..251

40. Pediatric Airway and Laryngeal Problems.................253
     Answers and Discussion..256

41. Facial Plastic Surgery...258
     Answers and Discussion..263

42. Head and Neck Reconstructive Surgery.....................266
     Answers and Discussion..269

43. Anesthesia for Head and Neck Surgery 271
     Answers and Discussion..274

44. Head and Neck Radiology..276
     Answers and Discussion..285

45. Pharmacology and Therapeutics 287
     Answers and Discussion..290

46. Miscellaneous Information..292
     Answers and Discussion..297

Preface

Otolaryngology—Head and Neck Surgery Specialty Board Review is intended to be a study guide for candidates preparing for the specialty board exams. This book is not a comprehensive manual but should be used to identify areas the candidate can concentrate on in preparing for the exams.

Introduction

Otolaryngology—Head and Neck Surgery Specialty Board Review is a concise question and answer review with detailed explanations and exact page references to K.J. Lee's *Essential Otolaryngology,* 6th Edition. The Table of Contents is arranged to correlate with *Essential Otolaryngology* to facilitate using the two books together for a comprehensive review for the certification examination. However, this review is complete enough that it can be used alone to provide a quick review.

Along with the references to *Essential Otolaryngology,* 6th Edition, there are other important textbooks referenced with exact pages. A list is provided on page xv.

The information is presented as 630 exact exam-type questions that follow the content outline for the certification examination. These items are similar both in scope and format to those you will encounter on the test to provide realistic practice sessions. The questions, and answers with explanations are in separate areas to allow you to test through an entire chapter before reviewing your answers. Once you have completed a section, you can move to the explanation section and quantify your results. This will provide you with a survey of your strengths and weaknesses and, thus, a road map for further study.

References

1. Lee KJ, ed. *Essential Otolaryngology.* 6th ed. Norwalk, CT: Appleton & Lange, 1995
2. Krause CJ, Pastorek N, Mangat DS, eds. *Aesthetic Facial Surgery.* Philadelphia: Lippincott, 1991
3. Bluestone CD, Stool SE, Scheetz MD, eds. *Pediatric Otolaryngology, Volumes I and II.* 2nd ed. Philadelphia: Saunders: 1990
4. Cummings CW, Krause CJ, Schuller DE, Fredrickson JM, Harker LE. *Otolaryngology—Head and Neck Surgery, Volumes I–IV.* 2nd ed. St Louis: Mosby, 1993

1

Anatomy of the Ear

1. The temporalis muscle attaches to the
   A. mastoid process
   B. tympanic portion of the temporal bone
   C. styloid process
   D. squamosa portion of the temporal bone
   E. greater wing of the sphenoid bone

2. The anterior boundary of the tympanic cavity is the
   A. styloid process, carotid wall
   B. styloid process, tensor palati
   C. carotid wall, tympanic part of the temporal bone
   D. eustachian tube, carotid wall, pyramidal prominence
   E. carotid wall, eustachian tube, tensor tympani

3. The Meckel cave (where the gasserian ganglion [V] is located) is a concavity in the following part of the temporal bone.
   A. anterior
   B. superior
   C. lateral
   D. medial
   E. anterior lateral

4. Gradenigo syndrome is associated with inflammation of the following cranial nerve in the Dorello canal.
   A. IV
   B. V
   C. VII
   D. VI
   E. III

5. Trautmann triangle is determined by the
   A. middle fossa dura plate, sigmoid sinus, and semicircular canals
   B. spine of Henle, dura plate, and semicircular canals
   C. sigmoid sinus, bony labyrinth, and superior petrosal sinus or dura
   D. bony labyrinth, spine of Henle, and semicircular canals
   E. lateral wall of epitympanum, dura plate, and sigmoid sinus

6. The upper limit of normal for the diameter of the internal auditory canal in an adult male is
   A. 9 mm
   B. 6 mm
   C. 7 mm
   D. 5 mm
   E. 8 mm

7. The posterior semicircular canal and saccule are innervated by the
   A. Jacobson nerve
   B. auricular temporal nerve
   C. inferior vestibular nerve
   D. auricular nerve
   E. superior vestibular nerve

8. The inferior tympanic artery to the middle ear is a branch of the
   A. postauricular artery
   B. caroticotympanic artery
   C. ascending pharyngeal artery
   D. external maxillary artery
   E. middle meningeal artery

9. The superior portions of the utricle and saccule and the superior and horizontal semicircular canals are supplied by the following artery
   A. anterior vestibular
   B. common cochlear
   C. cochlear vestibular
   D. posterior vestibular
   E. common cochlear

10. The lobule of the ear has sensory innervation from
    A. C_3 via the greater auricular nerve
    B. V_3 auricular temporal nerve
    C. X auricular branch
    D. VII auricular sensory nerve
    E. $C_{2,3}$ via lesser occipital nerve

11. The average size of the footplate is
    A. 1.41×2.99 mm
    B. 2.55×4.11 mm
    C. 1.22×2.13 mm
    D. 1.30×1.75 mm
    E. 3.00×3.75 mm

12. The scala vestibuli and the scala media are separated by the
    A. Reissner membrane
    B. tectorial membrane
    C. basilar membrane
    D. spiral ligament
    E. Deiters membrane

13. In the adult, the eustachian tube is approximately the following length
    A. 50 mm
    B. 20 mm
    C. 35 mm
    D. 40 mm
    E. 45 mm

14. The auricle of the ear has reached adult shape by the following week of gestation
    A. 8th
    B. 24th
    C. 20th
    D. 10th
    E. 30th

15. Congenital microtia occurs in the following incidence
    A. 1:20,000
    B. 1:50,000
    C. 1:40,000
    D. 1:100,000
    E. 1:60,000

Anatomy of the Ear

ANSWERS AND DISCUSSION

1. **(D)** This is important to know in performing a temporalis transfer procedure. The trigeminal nerve innervates from the undersurface, and the fan-shaped upper aspect provides good muscle body for facial reinnervation. (**Ref:** *Otolaryngology—Head and Neck Surgery,* **p. 1097**)

2. **(E)** This is important to be aware of in performing middle ear surgery, but it is also important clinically to appreciate the close proximity of the carotid artery in relationship to the middle ear. A patient with pulsatile tinnitus should be investigated from the point of view of any carotid abnormalities. (**Ref:** *Essential Otolaryngology,* **p. 2**)

3. **(B)** This is important, as this area can be the trigger site in someone with trigeminal neuralgia. (**Ref:** *Otolaryngology—Head and Neck Surgery,* **p. 1449**)

4. **(D)** The Dorello canal is between the petrous tip and the sphenoid bone. Gradenigo syndrome is related to petrositis in the ear with involvement of the VI nerve and is associated with pain behind the eye, diplopia, and aural discharge. (**Ref:** *Essential Otolaryngology,* **p. 3**)

5. **(C)** This is important because in mastoid surgery there is a very close relationship between the sigmoid sinus, the superior pet-

rosal sinus, and the bony labyrinth. (**Ref:** *Essential Otolaryngology*, **p. 3**)

6. **(E)** Acoustic neuromas can cause a widening of the internal auditory canal if they are associated with the nerve in the canal or at the cerebral pontine angle. (**Ref:** *Essential Otolaryngology*, **p. 4**)

7. **(C)** Surgical intervention in patients with persistent BPV or recurrent vestibulopathy involves singular neurectomy, vestibular neurectomy, and most recently posterior semicircular canal occlusion. (**Ref:** *Otolaryngology—Head and Neck Surgery*, **p. 3166**)

8. **(C)** The arterial supply to the middle ear is very generous and has blood supply from both the external and internal carotid artery. The long process of the incus receives the least blood supply and is most frequently necrosed. (**Ref:** *Essential Otolaryngology*, **p. 6**)

9. **(A)** A branch from the anterior vestibular artery forms the cochlear vestibular artery. The posterior vestibular artery supplies the inferior portion of the utricle and saccule and the posterior semicircular canal. (**Ref:** *Essential Otolaryngology*, **p. 7**)

10. **(E)** This nerve can be severed while doing a rhytidectomy and it is important to explain to a patient preoperatively that there may be some numbness to the ear lobe after surgery. (**Ref:** *Essential Otolaryngology*, **p. 7**)

11. **(A)** The size and thickness of the footplate are important in otosclerosis surgery. (**Ref:** *Essential Otolaryngology*, **p. 9**)

12. **(A)** The Reissner membrane is a three-layered structure, consisting of two cell layers separated by a basal lamina. The Reissner membrane is attached medially to the modiolar edge of the spiral limbus and laterally to the spiral ligament at the apical edge of the stria vascularis. (**Ref:** *Otolaryngology—Head and Neck Surgery*, **pp. 2499–2502**)

13. **(C)** At birth, the eustachian tube is horizontal and it grows to be on an incline of 45° in adult life. It is divided into an anteromedial cartilagious portion (24 mm) and a posterolateral bony por-

tion (11 mm). The narrowest part of the tube is at the junction of the bony and the cartilaginous portions. (**Ref:** *Essential Otolaryngology*, **p. 10)**

14. **(C)** This is important in congenital deformities of the ear. The majority of congenital deformities of the external ear occur around 12 weeks gestation or shortly thereafter. (**Ref:** *Essential Otolaryngology*, **p. 12)**

15. **(A)** Recessive microtia, meatal atresia, and hearing loss are autosomal recessive disorders. Anomalies of the external and middle ear include microtia, atresia of the external auditory canal, and malformed ossicles. (**Ref:** *Pediatric Otolaryngology*, **p. 286)**

2

Audiology

DIRECTIONS (Questions 16 through 35): Each of the numbered items or incomplete statements in this section is followed by answers or completions of the statement. Select the ONE lettered answer or completion that is BEST in each case.

16. The human ear is capable of hearing the frequency range from
    A. 500 to 5000 Hz
    B. 100 to 10,000 Hz
    C. 10 to 30,000 Hz
    D. 1000 to 10,000 Hz
    E. 20 to 20,000 Hz

17. In audiology, speech noise is white noise with the following frequencies filtered out
    A. below 300 Hz and above 3000 Hz
    B. below 800 Hz and above 4000 Hz
    C. below 100 Hz and above 5000 Hz
    D. below 50 Hz and above 8000 Hz
    E. below 20 Hz and above 20,000 Hz

18. The decibel scale is logarithmic and incorporates a ratio. All of the following are used for reference levels except
    A. intensity
    B. barometric pressure
    C. sound pressure
    D. hearing
    E. sensation level

19. The effective vibrating part of the tympanic membrane is approximately
    A. 90 mm^2
    B. 80 mm^2
    C. 70 mm^2
    D. 55 mm^2
    E. 40 mm^2

20. The transformer ratio of the middle ear is about 22:1. This translates into approximately
    A. 5 dB
    B. 10 dB
    C. 20 dB
    D. 25 dB
    E. 40 dB

21. In 1960, Bekesy outlined his theory of hearing. He stated that when the stapes footplate moves in and out of the oval window, there is a resulting upward and downward movement of the basilar membrane, which causes distortion of the endolymph. This theory is called the
    A. Resonance Theory of Hearing
    B. Place Theory of Hearing
    C. Traveling Wave Theory of Hearing
    D. Frequency Theory of Hearing
    E. Volley Theory of Hearing

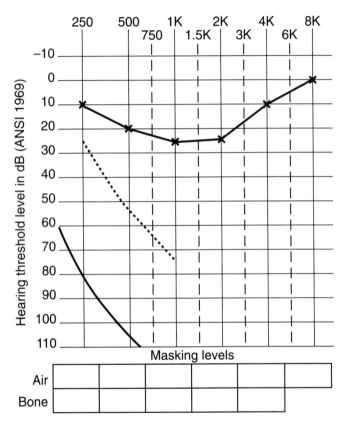

RIGHT EAR
Frequency in Hertz

22. The above audiogram is saucer shaped. This is most indicative of a
A. noise-induced hearing loss
B. tympanic membrane perforation
C. congenital hearing loss
D. presbyacusis
E. variant of normal hearing

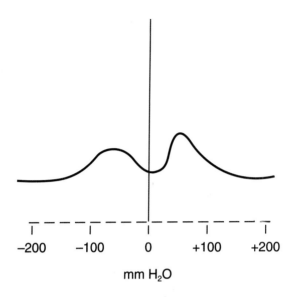

23. This impedance audiometry pattern can be seen in
    A. ossicular discontinuity
    B. the use of a high frequency probe tone in a "B" tympanogram
    C. barotrauma
    D. tympanic membrane perforation
    E. otitis media

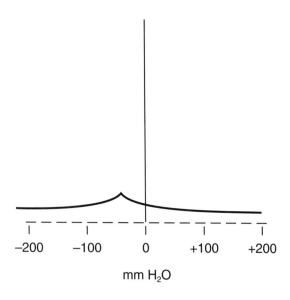

mm H$_2$O

24. This type of tympanogram is consistent with
   A. otosclerosis
   B. ossicular discontinuity
   C. serous otitis media
   D. barotrauma
   E. bullous myringitis

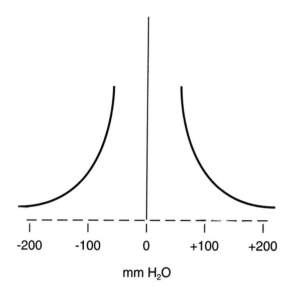

mm H$_2$O

25. The above tympanogram is a
    A. type A
    B. type B
    C. type C
    D. type A$_s$
    E. type A$_d$

26. During a Carhart Tone Decay Test, one presents a tone at the threshold for the following number of seconds
    A. 20
    B. 40
    C. 60
    D. 80
    E. 90

27. The following test is similar to the Carhart test but it incorporates rest periods during the testing. It is the
    A. Olson–Noffsinger Test
    B. Owen Test
    C. Rosenberg One-Minute Test
    D. Green Modified Tone Decay Test
    E. Suprathreshold Adaptation Test

28. In Bekesy Audiometry when there is a continuous tracing above the pulsed tracing, this is indicative of a functional hearing loss. This is called a Bekesy type
    A. I
    B. II
    C. III
    D. IV
    E. V

29. In acoustic reflex testing, the reflex will likely be absent if there is conductive pathology or a sensorineural hearing loss greater than
    A. 20 dB
    B. 40 dB
    C. 60 dB
    D. 70 dB
    E. 80 dB

30. In high risk neonates, the following percentage of the screen group will have hearing loss using Brainstem Evoked Response Audiometry
    A. 1 to 2%
    B. 2 to 3%
    C. 3 to 4%
    D. 5 to 7%
    E. > 7%

31. The audiometric test that is based on the principle that one increases the volume of one's voice in the presence of background noise due to the fact that the noise is heard and interferes with self-monitoring is called the
    A. Lombard Test
    B. Stenger Test
    C. Doerfler–Stewart Test
    D. Griesinger Test
    E. Steward Test

32. A positive Bing test is indicative of
    A. conductive hearing loss
    B. tympanic membrane perforation
    C. normal hearing

D. sensorineural hearing loss
E. mixed hearing loss

33. The tuning fork test in which the tuning fork is placed against the mastoid and then, when it is no longer heard, is placed against the tragus while the examiner gently occludes the meatus is called the
   A. Lewis Test
   B. Gelle Test
   C. Schwabach Test
   D. Bing Test
   E. Weber Test

34. According to OSHA, Permissible Noise Exposure over an 8-hour day should not exceed
   A. 70 dB
   B. 80 dB
   C. 90 dB
   D. 100 dB
   E. 110 dB

35. Earmuffs, custom-fitted earplugs, or disposable earplugs each provide the following amount of sound attenuation
   A. 5 to 10 dB
   B. 10 to 20 dB
   C. 20 to 40 dB
   D. 40 to 50 dB
   E. 50 to 70 dB

Audiology

ANSWERS AND DISCUSSION

16. **(E)** Frequency refers to the number of cycles (complete oscillations) of a vibrating body per unit of time; the psychoacoustic equivalent of frequency is pitch. The human ear has the capability of hearing from approximately 20 to 20,000 Hz. (**Ref:** *Pediatric Otolaryngology,* **p. 88**)

17. **(A)** In audiology, white noise contains all frequencies in the spectrum. With speech noise, frequencies above 3000 Hz and below 300 Hz are filtered out. (**Ref:** *Essential Otolaryngology,* **p. 26**)

18. **(B)** Barometric pressure is incorrect. All the other factors are important, and it is important to remember a decibel is a logarithm of a ratio of two numbers or sounds: a referent and the sound being described. (**Ref:** *Essential Otolaryngology,* **p. 26**)

19. **(D)** Although the area of the tympanic membrane is 85 to 90 mm^2, only about 55 mm^2 effectively vibrates. (**Ref:** *Essential Otolaryngology,* **p. 29**)

20. **(D)** The result of the area effect of the tympanic membrane is 17:1 (the ratio of the vibrating portion of the tympanic membrane to that of the stapes footplate). The lever action of the ossicles is 1:3:1, therefore the transformer ratio is 22:1. (**Ref:** *Essential Otolaryngology,* **p. 29**)

21. (C) This is called the Traveling Wave Theory of Hearing. Current belief is that we hear by a combination of the above mechanisms. **(Ref: *Essential Otolaryngology*, p. 30)**

22. (C) This is indicative of a congenital hearing loss. **(Ref: *Essential Otolaryngology*, p. 41)**

23. (B) The notched tympanogram can be a result of a high frequency probe tone in the B-type tympanogram or the Y tympanogram in a normal ear. **(Ref: *Pediatric Otolaryngology*, p. 140)**

24. (A) This type of pattern can also be seen with otosclerosis or a scarred tympanic membrane. **(Ref: *Pediatric Otolaryngology*, p. 137)**

25. (E) This is consistent with disarticulation of the ossicular chain and indicates a "loose" middle ear system. **(Ref: *Pediatric Otolaryngology*, p. 137)**

26. (C) A tone is presented for 60 seconds in the Carhart Tone Decay Test. If the tone disappears, raise the stimulus level and continue until the patient can hear for 60 seconds. If this last level is 20 dB or more above threshold, the test is positive for retrocochlear pathology. **(Ref: *Essential Otolaryngology*, p. 48)**

27. (B) The Owen Test is a test to help rule out retrocochlear pathology. It is similar to the Carhart and Olson–Noffsinger Tests. **(Ref: *Essential Otolaryngology*, p. 48)**

28. (E) This is a Bekesy type V and it is important in distinguishing people who are malingering. **(Ref: *Essential Otolaryngology*, p. 49)**

29. (C) The acoustic reflex is usually absent if there is a greater than 60 dB sensorineural hearing loss. In normal hearing, stimulation of either side elicits a bilateral reflex. **(Ref: *Essential Otolaryngology*, p. 42)**

30. (C) Some of the criteria established by the Joint Committee on Infant Hearing include neonatal asphyxia, bacterial meningitis, congenital infection, defects of the head and neck, elevated bilirubin, family history of hearing loss, and low birth weight (<1500 grams). If these children are screened, about 3.5% will have hearing impairment. (**Ref:** *Pediatric Otolaryngology*, **p. 148**)

31. **(A)** This is a test to help determine if a patient has a functional hearing loss. (**Ref:** *Essential Otolaryngology*, **p. 60**)

32. **(C)** A positive Bing test is indicative of normal hearing. It is a tuning fork test in which the tone is louder with the ear canal occluded. (**Ref:** *Essential Otolaryngology*, **p. 33**)

33. **(A)** This is the Lewis Test. This is not a good test, and interpretation of the test is neither simple nor consistent. (**Ref:** *Essential Otolaryngology*, **p. 34**)

34. **(C)** The maximal permissible limit for exposure to noise over an 8-hour period is 90 dB. If one increased the noise to 95 dB, then the maximal exposure period would be 4 hours. (**Ref:** *Otolaryngology—Head and Neck Surgery*, **p. 2897**)

35. **(C)** Most commercially available ear plugs will provide only 20 to 40 dB of sound attenuation. (**Ref:** *Essential Otolaryngology*, **p. 67**)

3

Electrical Response Audiometry

DIRECTIONS (Questions 36 through 45): Each of the numbered items or incomplete statements in this section is followed by answers or completions of the statement. Select the ONE lettered answer or completion that is BEST in each case.

---

36. The origin of the summating potential is the
   - **A.** hair cells
   - **B.** stria vascularis
   - **C.** auditory nerve
   - **D.** supporting cells
   - **E.** cochlear nucleus

37. The generator site for wave V of the brainstem evoked response audiometry (ABR) is thought to be the
   - **A.** auditory nerve
   - **B.** superior olive
   - **C.** inferior colliculus
   - **D.** hair cells
   - **E.** cochlear nucleus

38. The ABR generated by a broad-band click stimulus has its major contribution from the following frequency range
   A. 250 to 500 Hz
   B. 500 to 1000 Hz
   C. 1000 to 2000 Hz
   D. 2000 to 3000 Hz
   E. 3000 to 4000 Hz

39. A patient has a 60 dB hearing level at 4000 Hz in the suspect ear. To correct the latency of the ABR for this patient, the following time interval should be deducted
   A. 0.05 msec
   B. 0.1 msec
   C. 0.2 msec
   D. 0.3 msec
   E. 0.4 msec

40. The least interaural latency difference considered suspicious for an acoustic tumor is
   A. 0.1 msec
   B. 0.2 msec
   C. 0.3 msec
   D. 0.4 msec
   E. 0.5 msec

41. The cochlear microphonic originates from the
   A. auditory nerve
   B. cochlear nucleus
   C. stria vascularis
   D. hair cells
   E. inferior colliculus

42. Of the following, the most accurate noninvasive test for acoustic tumor diagnosis is
   A. computerized tomography
   B. auditory brainstem responses
   C. the crossed acoustic reflex
   D. temporal bone polytomography
   E. electronystagmosgraphy

43. The normal latency of the fifth wave of the ABR is in the range of
  A. 1 to 2 msec
  B. 2 to 3 msec
  C. 3 to 4 msec
  D. 4 to 5 msec
  E. 5 to 6 msec

44. The origin of wave I of the ABR is the
  A. primary auditory projections
  B. hair cells
  C. inferior colliculus
  D. auditory nerve
  E. cochlear nucleus

45. The normal value for the wave III–V interval is approximately
  A. 1 msec
  B. 2 msec
  C. 3 msec
  D. 4 msec

Electrical Response Audiometry

ANSWERS AND DISCUSSION

36. **(A)** The summating potential (SP) is generated by the hair cells and is a direct current shift of the baseline of the recording. It is almost always negative for all frequencies and intensity levels. (**Ref:** *Essential Otolaryngology,* **p. 76**)

37. **(C)** Wave II is from the VIIIth nerve or cochlear nucleus (3.0 msec). Wave III is the cochlear nucleus or superior olive (4.1 msec). Wave IV is the lateral lemniscus (5.3 msec). Wave V is the inferior colliculus (5.9 msec). (**Ref:** *Essential Otolaryngology,* **p. 73**)

38. **(E)** Generally, the accuracy below 3000 Hz is good but at high stimulus intensities much of the cochlea can be activated by tone bursts and correlations of responses to audiograms may be problematic. (**Ref:** *Essential Otolaryngology,* **p. 78**)

39. **(B)** For responses to a standard 80 dB nHL broadband click, we deduct 0.1 milliseconds for each 10 dB that the 4 kHz hearing loss exceeds 50 dB. This adjustment does not increase the number of false-negative results. (**Ref:** *Essential Otolaryngology,* **p. 85**)

40. (B) The interaural difference in wave V latency, called IT5, will normally be 0.2 milliseconds (allowing for observational error). Experience has shown that IT5 is greater than 0.2 milliseconds in more than 96% of acoustic tumors and thus is an excellent diagnostic measure. **(Ref: *Essential Otolaryngology*, p. 84)**

41. (D) The source of the cochlear microphonic (CM) is the hair-bearing surface of the hair cells. Its onset is immediate and it mimics the wave form of the acoustic stimulus. **(Ref: *Essential Otolaryngology*, p. 75)**

42. (B) The success of ABR depends on the fact that acoustic tumors stretch or compress the auditory nerve, producing a delay in the response latency that ABR can detect. This delay may occur in an ear with normal hearing. Conversely, cochlear lesions have little effect on the brainstem response latencies for high intensity stimuli until the hearing loss becomes severe. **(Ref: *Essential Otolaryngology*, p. 84)**

43. (E) Wave V is at the level of the inferior colliculus and has a normal latency of 5.9 msec. **(Ref: *Essential Otolaryngology*, p. 73)**

44. (D) Wave I has a normal latency of 2.0 msec. **(Ref: *Essential Otolaryngology*, p. 73)**

45. (B) Normally, wave III latency is 4.1 msec and wave V latency is 5.9 msec. Any prolongation of the wave III–V interval over 1.8 msec is suspicious of a possible acoustic neuroma. **(Ref: *Essential Otolaryngology*, p. 73)**

4

The Vestibular System and Its Disorders, Part I

DIRECTIONS (Questions 46 through 55): Each of the numbered items or incomplete statements in this section is followed by answers or completions of the statement. Select the ONE lettered answer or completion that is BEST in each case.

---

46. The kinocilia are located
- **A.** in the saccule
- **B.** in the utricle
- **C.** completely along the top of each hair cell
- **D.** at the end of each hair cell nearest the tallest stereocilia
- **E.** in the saccular aqueduct

47. The utricle is primarily sensitive to
- **A.** vertical movement
- **B.** angular movement
- **C.** circular movement
- **D.** linear movement
- **E.** spatial movement

48. A 40-year-old patient is having a caloric test done. Stimulating the right ear with water warmer than body temperature results in the following directional movement of endolymph
  A. ampullofugal
  B. vertical
  C. utriculofugal
  D. away from the utricle
  E. ampullopetal

49. The endolymphatic potential across the membrane separating the endolymph from the perilymph is
  A. 20 mV
  B. 40 mV
  C. 80 mV
  D. 200 mV
  E. 150 mV

50. In electronystagmography testing (ENG), investigators use the following percentage difference between right-beating and left-beating nystagmus to be significant in the Jongkee formula for directional preponderance (DP)
  A. 10 to 15%
  B. 15 to 20%
  C. 25 to 30%
  D. 35 to 40%
  E. 40 to 45%

51. A 50-year-old male presents with vertigo. During his ENG testing, he has a right-beating nystagmus with the left ear down and a left-beating nystagmus with the right ear down. This is suspicious of
  A. multiple sclerosis
  B. viral labyrinthitis
  C. positional alcohol nystagmus
  D. benign positional vertigo
  E. Ménière disease

52. Simultaneous binaural bithermal stimulus testing produces diagnostic information and is what percentage more sensitive than the alternate binaural bithermal method done?
    A. 10%
    B. 20%
    C. 30%
    D. 45%
    E. 55%

53. A 60-year-old male is suspected of having a central lesion. One of the most reliable signs would be
    A. failure of ocular fixation
    B. right-beating nystagmus
    C. direction-fixed nystagmus
    D. direction-changing position nystagmus
    E. ocular fixation

54. Alternate bithermal caloric responses may reveal an abnormality about 50% of the time while simultaneous bithermal caloric responses increase the yield to 80% in the following condition
    A. vestibular neuritis
    B. Ménière disease
    C. acoustic neuroma
    D. perilymph fistula
    E. multiple sclerosis

55. On ENG testing of a 23-year-old female with symptoms of unsteadiness, it was noted that there was evidence of anterior internuclear ophthalmoplegia on testing eye movements. This is indicative of
    A. acoustic neuroma
    B. Ménière syndrome
    C. subarachnoid hemorrhage
    D. syphilis
    E. multiple sclerosis

The Vestibular System and Its Disorders, Part I

ANSWERS AND DISCUSSION

46. (D) Each hair cell has two varieties of hairs or cilia. The stereocilia are arranged in an ascending pipe organ manner. A single kinocilium is located at the end nearest the tallest stereocilia. The kinocilium is less rigid in structure than the stereocilia and appears wavy and more flexible. The deflection of the cilia either toward or away from the kinocilium stimulates the hair cell. (**Ref:** *Essential Otolaryngology*, **p. 94**)

47. (D) The utricle is the primary otolithic structure sensitive to linear acceleration. The function of the saccule is not clear. It may function similarly to the utricle and/or as a low frequency sound or vibration sensor. (**Ref:** *Essential Otolaryngology*, **p. 93**)

48. (E) Stimulating the right ear with water warmer than the body temperature results in an ampullopetal (toward the ampulla) or utriculopetal (toward the utricle) movement of endolymph. This endolymph flow deflects the stereocilia toward the kinocilia. (**Ref:** *Essential Otolaryngology*, **p. 94**)

49. (C) The endolymph potassium is at intracellular concentration. To maintain this 80 mV potential, a glucose–metabolism-based high energy output is used. (**Ref: *Essential Otolaryngology,* p. 94**)

50. **(C)** Directional preponderance (DP) refers only to bithermal caloric testing. It simply means there is more nystagmus beating in one direction compared to the other despite normal differences between ears. When present at pathologic or significant levels, it means that the vestibular system is not functioning normally and is not useful for localizing the disorder. (**Ref: *Essential Otolaryngology,* p. 102**)

51. **(C)** The cupula is rendered a floating object by alcohol diffusion. It becomes gravity dependent and produces a peripheral vestibular abnormality secondary to the prior 24- to 48-hour ingestion of alcohol. The patient must be carefully questioned regarding the ingestion of substances that could alter the vestibular evaluation. (**Ref: *Essential Otolaryngology,* p. 102**)

52. **(E)** For this reason, simultaneous binaural bithermal stimulus is recommended as a 6.5-minute addition to the vestibular evaluation. (**Ref: *Essential Otolaryngology,* pp. 103–104**)

53. **(A)** Failure of ocular fixation suppression is a very reliable sign of a central disorder. (**Ref: *Essential Otolaryngology,* p. 104**)

54. **(B)** The ENG testing in Ménière disease commonly shows very little between the initial episodes. During attacks, there may be active spontaneous nystagmus with direction-changing components even in the midst of caloric testing. (**Ref: *Essential Otolaryngology,* pp. 108–109**)

55. **(E)** ENG in multiple sclerosis may show anything from normal or peripheral or central findings. Auditory brainstem evoked potentials may show delay of central conduction. More likely, usually evoked potentials are significantly delayed. Internuclear ophthalmoplegia is almost pathognomonic of multiple sclerosis. (**Ref: *Essential Otolaryngology,* p. 108**)

5

The Vestibular System and Its Disorders, Part II

DIRECTIONS (Questions 56 through 65): Each of the numbered items or incomplete statements in this section is followed by answers or completions of the statement. Select the ONE lettered answer or completion that is BEST in each case.

56. Nystagmus present when gazing in the direction of the fast component and in straight gaze is termed
    A. first-degree spontaneous nystagmus
    B. positional nystagmus
    C. Aschan type II nystagmus
    D. second-degree nystagmus
    E. Nylen type I nystagmus

57. Positional nystagmus, when the direction of the nystagmus remains fixed regardless of the position of the head during the positional testing although it may be stronger in a particular direction, is termed
    A. Nylen type II nystagmus
    B. second-degree nystagmus
    C. third-degree nystagmus
    D. Nylen type III nystagmus
    E. Nylen type I nystagmus

58. Aschan type I nystagmus is when
  A. the direction of nystagmus varies with the head during positional testing
  B. the nystagmus is present when gazing in the direction of the first component and on straight gaze
  C. the nystagmus is nonfatigable and persistent: its direction remains fixed with change of head position
  D. the nystagmus is nonfatigable and persistent: its direction changes with head position
  E. the nystagmus is present only when gazing in the direction of the first component

59. The Kobrak test is a simple caloric test that is done with the patient in the upright position and the head tilted back at a
  A. 90° angle
  B. 30° angle
  C. 60° angle
  D. 45° angle
  E. 15° angle

60. The directional preponderance test is a standardized test to measure canal paresis and directional preponderance and in this test the patient is placed supine and the head is elevated at a
  A. 15° angle
  B. 30° angle
  C. 45° angle
  D. 60° angle
  E. 0° angle

61. The principle of electronystagmography is based on the difference in electrical potential between the retina (–) and the
  A. skin over the eyelid
  B. skin over forehead
  C. lens
  D. cornea
  E. tarsal plate

62. In a positive fistula test, stimulation of the ear with positive pressure results in nystagmus
   A. to the same side
   B. to the opposite side
   C. in a vertical direction
   D. in a rotary direction
   E. in a variable direction

63. The Charcot triad (nystagmus, scanning speech, intention tremor) may be associated with
   A. multiple sclerosis
   B. Parkinson disease
   C. congenital syphilis
   D. basilar–vertebral insufficiency
   E. Wallenberg syndrome

64. The rare variant of Ménière disease in which there is a dramatic restoration of hearing after an acute attack of vertigo is called
   A. crises of Tumarkin
   B. Cogan syndrome
   C. Lermoyez syndrome
   D. Rollet syndrome
   E. Shafer syndrome

65. Internuclear ophthalmoplegia is a disturbance of the lateral movements of the eyes characterized by a paralysis of the internal rectus on one side and weakness of the external rectus on the other, and if it is bilateral it is pathognomonic of
   A. myasthenia gravis
   B. Cogan syndrome
   C. congenital syphilis
   D. Wallenberg syndrome
   E. multiple sclerosis

The Vestibular System and Its Disorders, Part II

ANSWERS AND DISCUSSION

56. (D) Second-degree spontaneous nystagmus suggests a central origin. Also, vertical or diagonal nystagmus suggests a central origin. (**Ref:** *Essential Otolaryngology,* **p. 98**)

57. (A) This implies either a peripheral lesion or a central lesion such as an acoustic neuroma. Nylen type I nystagmus is when the direction of the nystagmus varies with the position of the head during positional testing and implies a central lesion. (**Ref:** *Essential Otolaryngology,* **p. 98**)

58. (D) This indicates a CNS etiology. Aschan type II nystagmus is different from type I in that its direction remains fixed with change in head position. This is mainly associated with CNS disorders. Type III is all varieties of transitory positional nystagmus with latency and fatigue. This is associated with peripheral disease. (**Ref:** *Essential Otolaryngology,* **p. 98**)

59. (C) The Kobrak Test is used to measure the latency and duration of nystagmus. One uses 0.2 to 5.0 mL of ice water instilled against the tympanic membrane with the patient in a sitting position and the head tilted back 60°. (**Ref:** *Essential Otolaryngology,* **p. 100**)

60. (B) In this test, each ear is douched in turn with no less than 250 mL of water at 86° F (30° C) and 112° F (44° C). At least 5 minutes must elapse between each douche. Directional preponderance is believed to be toward the side of a central lesion and away from the side of a peripheral lesion. **(Ref: *Essential Otolaryngology*, p. 103)**

61. (D) During the nystagmus, movements of the eyes cause this corneal–retinal potential to be displaced laterally, giving rise to changes in potential that can be recorded by electronic equipment. This electronic recording of the nystagmus is the ENG value. **(Ref: *Essential Otolaryngology*, pp. 100–101)**

62. (A) An inner ear fistula is defined as an abnormal communication between the perilymphatic space and the middle ear or an intramembraneous communication between endolymphatic and perilymphatic spaces. If there is a positive fistula sign, surgical exploration is recommended. **(Ref: *Otolaryngology—Head and Neck Surgery*, pp. 3167–3168)**

63. (A) Vertigo can be the presenting symptom in 10% of multiple sclerosis patients. There is an increased gamma globulin level in the CSF in 90% of these patients and, on MRI scan in 70 to 95% of patients, one may identify white matter lesions. **(Ref: *Essential Otolaryngology*, p. 110)**

64. (C) This is a rare presentation of Ménière disease. There is an increased tinnitus and hearing loss before the episode with a dramatic resolution after the episode. The crises of Tumarkin is a sudden unexplained fall without loss of consciousness. It is felt that this is a consequence of an abrupt change in otolithic input. **(Ref: *Otolaryngology—Head and Neck Surgery*, p. 3157)**

65. (E) Blurring or loss of vision caused by demyelinating of the optic nerve (retrobulbar neuritis) is the initial symptom of multiple sclerosis in approximately 20% of patients. Hearing loss occurs in approximately 25% of patients. **(Ref: *Otolaryngology—Head and Neck Surgery*, pp. 3192–3193)**

6

Speech, Language, and Voice

DIRECTIONS (Questions 66 through 75): Each of the numbered items or incomplete statements in this section is followed by answers or completions of the statement. Select the ONE lettered answer or completion that is BEST in each case.

---

66. A speech impairment that occurs with a cerebrovascular accident or another neurologic problem in which substitutions and additions of sounds in words is termed
    A. apraxia
    B. dysarthria
    C. dysfluency
    D. misarticulation
    E. disarticulation

67. When a child tends to repeat what is said to him or her it is termed
    A. echolalia
    B. repetitive verbal child
    C. aphasia
    D. multiple aphasia
    E. dysphasia

68. The frequency of voice that is considered optimal for adult men is at
    A. 75 Hz
    B. 125 Hz
    C. 200 Hz
    D. 250 Hz
    E. 500 Hz

69. A 40-year-old male presents to his physician with a voice disorder. He is diagnosed as having flaccid dysarthria. His most likely diagnosis contributing to this is
    A. myasthenia gravis
    B. multiple sclerosis
    C. Parkinson disease
    D. amyotrophic lateral sclerosis
    E. alcohol intoxication

70. Amyotrophic lateral sclerosis is a condition in which a voice disorder may present as
    A. flaccid dysarthria
    B. spastic dysarthria
    C. atoxic dysarthria
    D. hypokinetic dysarthria
    E. mixed dysarthria

71. One of the most important tests in detecting vibratory assymmetries and submucosal scars is
    A. ultra-high speed photography
    B. electroglottography
    C. strobovideolaryngoscopy
    D. ultrasound glottography
    E. photoelectroglottography

72. The region of the intermediate and deep layers of the lamina propria is called the
    A. Reinkes space
    B. vocal ligament
    C. fibroblastic layer
    D. vocal fold
    E. membranous portion of the vocal fold

73. The volume of air remaining in the lungs at the end of expiration during normal breathing, which may be divided into expiratory reserve volume and residual volume, is called
   A. tidal volume
   B. functional residual capacity
   C. inspiratory capacity
   D. vital capacity
   E. forced vital capacity

74. This medication has been used in treatment of performance anxiety but can produce thrombocytopenic purpura, mental depression, and bronchospasm among other adverse reactions.
   A. ativan
   B. valium
   C. beta blockers
   D. alpha blockers
   E. cimetidine

75. The theory of speech that suggests that the contribution of a particular speech maneuver to the spectrum depends on its relation to the nodes or antinodes of the standing waves is called the
   A. perturbation theory
   B. quantal theory
   C. source filter theory
   D. linguistic theory
   E. motor theory

Speech, Language, and Voice

ANSWERS AND DISCUSSION

66. **(A)** This speech impairment is called apraxia. Dysarthria is a central or peripheral nervous system deficit resulting in muscle slowness, weakness, or incoordination. **(Ref:** *Essential Otolaryngology,* **p. 129)**

67. **(A)** This term is echolalia. **(Ref:** *Essential Otolaryngology,* **p. 129)**

68. **(B)** The frequency considered optimal for adult men is 125 Hz and for women is 225 Hz. **(Ref:** *Essential Otolaryngology,* **p. 135)**

69. **(A)** Flaccid dysarthria is a voice disorder that occurs in lower motor neuron or primary muscle disorders such as myasthenia gravis and tumors and strokes involving the brainstem nuclei. **(Ref:** *Otolaryngology—Head and Neck Surgery,* **p. 2042)**

70. **(E)** Mixed dysarthria occurs in amyotrophic lateral sclerosis. Ataxic dysarthria is seen with cerebellar disease, alcohol intoxication, and multiple sclerosis. **(Ref:** *Otolaryngology—Head and Neck Surgery,* **p. 2042)**

71. **(C)** Strobovideolaryngoscopy is one of the single most important technologic advances in diagnostic laryngology. It is useful in the patient who has poor voice quality after laryngeal surgery with a normal larynx on physical exam. **(Ref:** *Otolaryngology— Head and Neck Surgery,* **p. 2036)**

72. **(B)** This is called the vocal ligament. Reinkes space is the superficial layer of the lamina propria. **(Ref:** *Otolaryngology— Head and Neck Surgery,* **p. 2020)**

73. **(B)** Aerodynamic measures are very important in assessing the professional voice and this is the "power source" of the voice. **(Ref:** *Otolaryngology—Head and Neck Surgery,* **p. 2037)**

74. **(C)** Beta blockers have been used to help individuals with performance anxiety but can have many side effects including hypotension and so on. **(Ref:** *Otolaryngology—Head and Neck Surgery,* **p. 2043)**

75. **(A)** This is called the perturbation theory. In this theory, it is suggested that widening near a volume velocity node lowers the frequency of that resonance, while narrowing raises it. **(Ref:** *Otolaryngology—Head and Neck Surgery,* **p. 1743)**

7

Congenital Deafness

DIRECTIONS (Questions 76 through 100): Each of the numbered items or incomplete statements in this section is followed by answers or completions of the statement. Select the ONE lettered answer or completion that is BEST in each case.

---

76. Hereditary deafness occurs in the following incidence of live births
    A. 1:4000
    B. 1:10,000
    C. 1:20,000
    D. 1:2000
    E. 1:15,000

77. The Mundini–Alexander classification of inner ear developmental anomalies is
   A. membranous cochlea–saccular aplasia. The bony labyrinth is normal, as are the utricles and semicircular canals (pars superior).
   B. complete failure of development of the inner ear (bony and membranous).
   C. incomplete development of the bony and membranous labyrinth. The cochlea may be represented by a single curved tube and the vestibular labyrinth is not developed.
   D. partial aplasia of the cochlear duct giving rise to high frequency hearing loss.
   E. the membranous vestibular apparatus is maldeveloped. The membranous cochlea may or may not be normal.

78. If a mother is infected with rubella during the first trimester, the percentage of children with deafness at birth is
   A. < 5%
   B. 5 to 10%
   C. 15 to 20%
   D. 10 to 15%
   E. > 20%

79. In a congenital syphilis patient, when there is vertigo and nystagmus on stimulation with high intensity sound such as the Barany noise box, it is called a
   A. positive Hennebert sign
   B. positive Barany sign
   C. Tullio phenomenon
   D. positive Kernig sign
   E. positive Henderson sign

80. Leopard syndrome is a form of hereditary congenital deafness associated with variable sensorineural hearing loss, pulmonary stenosis, hypogonadism, and
   A. blue irides
   B. elevated sweat chlorides
   C. ocular hypertelorism
   D. small dystrophic nails
   E. mitral insufficiency

81. Tietze syndrome is a hereditary congenital deafness associated with profound deafness, absent eyebrows, blue irides, and
    A. uniform teeth
    B. brown spots on the skin
    C. abnormalities of the genitalia
    D. mental retardation
    E. albinism

82. The autosomal dominant hereditary congenital deafness syndrome associated with widely spaced medial canthi, flat nasal root in 75% of the cases, confluent eyebrows, white forelock, and colored irides is
    A. Forney syndrome
    B. ectodermal dysplasia
    C. Mohr syndrome
    D. Waardenburg disease
    E. Hunter syndrome

83. Achondroplasia is associated with saddle nose, frontal and mandibular prominence, mixed hearing loss, and
    A. dwarfism
    B. mitral insufficiency
    C. abnormal tyrosine metabolism
    D. confluent eyebrows
    E. fine retinal pigmentation

84. The hereditary congenital deafness syndrome associated with syndactylia, craniofacial dysostosis, hypoplastic maxilla, exophthalmos, and a flat conductive hearing loss is
    A. Mohr syndrome
    B. Forney syndrome
    C. Roaf syndrome
    D. Apert syndrome
    E. Baelz syndrome

85. The hereditary congenital deafness syndrome associated with cranial synostosis, parrot-beaked nose, short upper lip, mandibular prognathism, and premature closure of the cranial suture lines is
   A. Crouzon syndrome
   B. Hippel–Lindau syndrome
   C. Mohr syndrome
   D. Englemann syndrome
   E. Piebaldness syndrome

86. Klippel–Feil syndrome is a hereditary congenital deafness associated with sensorineural hearing loss, short neck due to fused cervical vertebrae, external auditory canal atresia, and
   A. congenital flexion contractures of fingers and toes
   B. hypoplastic maxilla
   C. spina bifida
   D. internal hydrocephalis
   E. cleft palate

87. The syndrome of congenital deafness, pigeon breast, scoliosis, thin elongated individuals with long spidery fingers and hammer toes is
   A. Sturge–Weber
   B. Tapia
   C. cleidocranial
   D. Englemann
   E. Marfan

88. A 6-month-old male presents with hearing loss, optic atrophy, sclerotic brittle bone, choanal atresia, and fluctuating facial nerve paralysis. The most likely diagnosis is
   A. Roaf syndrome
   B. Albers–Schonberg disease
   C. Klippel–Feil syndrome
   D. Pyle syndrome
   E. osteitis deformans

89. Treacher Collins syndrome is associated with malformation of ossicles, antimongoloid palpebral fissure, mandibular hypoplasia, and a
   A. normal IQ
   B. cleft palate

    C. preauricular fistula
    D. glossoptosis
    E. subglottic stenosis

90. A 1-year-old male presents with micrognathia, cleft palate, mixed hearing loss, hypoplastic mandible, mental retardation, and breathing difficulties when sleeping. The most likely diagnosis is
    A. Pyle syndrome
    B. Oto–palatal–digital syndrome
    C. Samters syndrome
    D. Van Buchem syndrome
    E. Pierre Robin syndrome

91. Van der Hoeve syndrome or osteogenesis imperfecta is an autosomal dominant congenital hearing loss syndrome associated with fragile bones, loose ligaments, hearing loss, and 60% have
    A. cleft lip and cleft palate
    B. mental retardation
    C. blue sclera
    D. retinal atrophy
    E. torticollis

92. Alport syndrome is suspected in a 4-month-old baby. One of the most helpful tests in making the diagnosis would be a
    A. peripheral blood smear
    B. bone marrow exam
    C. liver function screen
    D. urinalysis
    E. chest x-ray

93. Fanconi anemia syndrome, Alstrom syndrome, Van Buchem syndrome, and Mohr syndrome all share the same trait of
    A. autosomal recessive inheritance
    B. deformed thumb
    C. cranial nerve palsies
    D. retinal degeneration
    E. dwarfism

94. Hallgren syndrome, Alstrom syndrome, and Cockayne syndrome all share the same trait of
   A. autosomal dominant inheritance
   B. associated visual loss
   C. choanal atresia
   D. hypoplastic mandible
   E. micrognathia

95. Hurler syndrome (gargoylism) is a hereditary congenital deafness syndrome associated with mental retardation, dwarfism, mixed hearing loss, forehead prominence, and
   A. progressive myopia and cataracts
   B. goiter
   C. abnormal development of the petrous pyramid
   D. hypogonadism
   E. abnormal mucopolysaccharides are deposited in tissues

96. Laurence–Moon–Bardet–Biedl syndrome is associated with congenital deafness, obesity, dwarfism, mental retardation, and
   A. retinitis pigmentosa
   B. pancytopenia
   C. increased skin pigmentation
   D. progressive ataxia
   E. diabetes mellitus

97. Pendred syndrome is a hereditary congenital deafness syndrome associated with a "U"-shaped audiogram, diffuse goiter developing at puberty, and a normal IQ. This syndrome constitutes the following percentage of hereditary deafness syndromes
   A. 20%
   B. 10%
   C. 5%
   D. 2%
   E. 15%

98. The syndrome associated with retinitis pigmentosa, polyneuropathy, ataxia, and sensorineural hearing loss is
   A. Norrie syndrome
   B. Richard–Rundel syndrome

C. Taylor syndrome
D. Refsum syndrome
E. Hallgren syndrome

99. With regards to congenital abnormalities of the middle and external ear, when one has microtia, atretic canals, and abnormal ossicles it is termed a
   A. class II abnormality
   B. class V abnormality
   C. class I abnormality
   D. class III abnormality
   E. class IV abnormality

100. The hereditary congenital deafness syndrome that is autosomal recessive and is associated with retinitis pigmentosa, ataxia, and vestibular dysfunction is
   A. Weil syndrome
   B. Möbius syndrome
   C. Hunter syndrome
   D. Usher syndrome
   E. Alstrom syndrome

Congenital Deafness

ANSWERS AND DISCUSSION

76. (A) One percent of hereditary deafness is sex linked, 9% is due to an autosomal dominant inheritance, and 90% is the result of autosomal recessive transmission. Dominant hearing loss usually progresses, whereas the recessive type is nonprogressive. (**Ref:** *Essential Otolaryngology,* **p. 143**)

77. (C) Michel is the complete failure of development of the inner ear (bony and membranous aplasia). The middle ear and external auditory canal may be normal. The Scheibe classification is such that there is membranous cochlea–saccular aplasia (pars inferior) but the bony labyrinth is normal, as are the utriculus and semicircular canals (pars superior). Alexander is partial aplasia of the cochlear duct giving rise to high frequency hearing loss, and Bing–Siebermann is maldeveloped membranous vestibular apparatus. (**Ref:** *Essential Otolaryngology,* **p. 143**)

78. (B) Maternal rubella manifestations include malleus and stapes abnormalities with cartilaginous fixation of the stapes footplate. Also there is depression of the Reissner membrane, hair cell degeneration, spiral ganglion loss, and collapse of the saccular membrane. Audiometric testing reveals sensorineural and conductive hearing losses. (**Ref:** *Otolaryngology—Head and Neck Surgery,* **p. 287**)

79. **(C)** This can also occur in congenital syphilis patients with a semicircular canal fistula and also in postfenestration patients if the footplate is mobile and in the fenestrum patient. **(Ref: *Essential Otolaryngology*, p. 145)**

80. **(C)** Blue irides is associated with piebaldness and Tietze syndrome. Forney syndrome is associated with mitral insufficiency, lentigines, skeletal abnormalities, and conductive hearing loss. **(Ref: *Essential Otolaryngology*, p. 146)**

81. **(E)** Also associated with this are blue irides, no photophobia or nystagmus, and profound deafness. It is autosomal dominant. **(Ref: *Essential Otolaryngology*, p. 147)**

82. **(D)** The two most common abnormalities in Waardenburg syndrome are dystrophic canthi and abnormal intercanthal distance. Histopathologic findings show a normal bony labyrinth, lack of the organ of corti and spiral ganglion cells, as well as atrophy of the stria vascularis. The vestibular labyrinth is normal. **(Ref: *Pediatric Otolaryngology*, pp. 550–551)**

83. **(A)** Achondroplasia is a hereditary dominant disorder. It occurs in 1 of 10,000 newborn infants and 1 of 50,000 of the general population. **(Ref: *Pediatric Otolaryngology*, p. 278)**

84. **(D)** Another name for Apert syndrome is acrocephalosyndactylia. It is an autosomal dominant trait. It occurs at a rate of 1 in 100,000 to 1 in 160,000. **(Ref: *Pediatric Otolaryngology*, p. 278)**

85. **(A)** Craniofacial dysostosis is a hereditary autosomal dominant disorder. Audiometric findings reveal that approximately one third of the patients with this syndrome have a hearing loss that is usually nonprogressive and conductive in nature. **(Ref: *Pediatric Otolaryngology*, p. 281)**

86. **(C)** Brevicollis or Klippel–Feil syndrome is a hereditary disorder that appears to be due to a recessive gene. Females are predominantly affected and the disease is rare. Deafness is the second most common finding in this disorder and is of the

sensorineural or mixed type. There is frequently an absence of vestibular function. (**Ref:** *Pediatric Otolaryngology*, **p. 279**)

87. (E) Marfan syndrome is an autosomal dominant disorder in which individuals have a tall stature with a disproportionately long lower segment, long fingers and toes, detached lens, and aortic aneurysms. (**Ref:** *Essential Otolaryngology*, **p. 149**)

88. (B) Marble bone disease, osteopetrosis, or Albers–Schonberg disease is of autosomal recessive inheritance. There is a conductive or mixed hearing loss. The bone is brittle due to failure of resorption of calcified cartilage. There may be involvement of cranial nerves II, V, and VII and there can be optic atrophy. (**Ref:** *Essential Otolaryngology*, **p. 149**)

89. (A) Mandibulofacial dysostolsis or Treacher Collins syndrome is of dominant inheritance. There is an absence of eyelashes medially, a short palate, and hypoplasia of the malar bones and intraorbital rims. (**Ref:** *Essential Otolaryngology*, **p. 151**)

90. (E) Pierre Robin syndrome is an autosomal dominant trait with variable penetrance. The prevalence is 1 in 30,000 live births. It may also result from an intrauterine insult. There may be associated hydrocephalus, microcephaly, myopia, retinal detachments, sixth nerve palsy, and congenital cataracts. (**Ref:** *Pediatric Otolaryngology*, **p. 280**)

91. (C) Osteogenesis imperfecta is a hereditary autosomal dominant disease. It is characterized by defective synthesis of connective tissue, including bone matrix. There is also abnormal tooth dentin with caries and dental fractures. The hearing loss is usually conductive in nature. (**Ref:** *Pediatric Otolaryngology*, **p. 285**)

92. (D) In Alport syndrome, the kidneys are affected by chronic glomerulonephritis with interstitial lymphocytic infiltrate and foam cells. Progressive sensorineural hearing loss begins at age 10. It affects all males but not all female subjects. This contributes to 1% of hereditary deafness. (**Ref:** *Essential Otolaryngology*, **p. 152**)

93. **(A)** Fanconi anemia syndrome is associated with an absent or deformed thumb. Hurler syndrome is associated with dwarfism. Cockayne syndrome is associated with retinal degeneration and osteopetrosis is associated with cranial nerve palsies. **(Ref: *Essential Otolaryngology*, pp. 154–155)**

94. **(B)** Alstrom syndrome is also associated with diabetes, obesity, and progressive sensorineural hearing loss. Hallgren syndrome is also associated with progressive ataxia, mental retardation, sensorineural hearing loss, and as well constitutes 5% of hereditary deafness. Cockayne syndrome is associated with dwarfism, mental retardation, and motor disturbances. **(Ref: *Essential Otolaryngology*, p. 153)**

95. **(E)** In Hurler syndrome, there is also chondroitin sulfate B and hepartin in the urine, progressive corneal opacities, hepatosplenomegaly, and dwarfism. **(Ref: *Essential Otolaryngology*, pp. 154–155)**

96. **(A)** Laurence–Moon–Biedl syndrome is an autosomal recessive disease with also hypogonadism, retinitis pigmentosa, and sensorineural hearing loss. **(Ref: *Essential Otolaryngology*, p. 155)**

97. **(B)** Pendred syndrome is a very common cause of hereditary deafness. It is autosomal recessive. The goiter is treated with exogenous hormone to suppress thyroid-stimulating hormone (TSH) secretion. There is also a positive perchlorate test. **(Ref: *Essential Otolaryngology*, p. 156)**

98. **(D)** Refsum disease or heredopathia atactica polyneuritiformis is an autosomal recessive disease that also has associated sensorineural hearing loss, visual impairment usually beginning in the second decade, and elevated plasma phytanic acid levels. **(Ref: *Essential Otolaryngology*, pp. 156–157)**

99. **(D)** Class II abnormalities are associated with microtia, atretic canal, and abnormal ossicles with normal aeration of mastoid and middle ear. Class I abnormalities have a normal auricle in shape and size, a well-pneumatized mastoid and middle ear, an ossicular problem, and is the most common type. **(Ref: *Essential Otolaryngology*, p. 159)**

100. (D) Weil syndrome is associated with nephritis, hearing loss, and is autosomal dominant. Möbius syndrome or congenital facial diplegia is associated with facial diplegia, external ear deformities, ophthalmoplegia, and mental retardation. Hunter syndrome is the same as Hurler syndrome except that it is sex linked. (**Ref: Essential Otolaryngology, p. 159**)

8

Cochlear Implants

DIRECTIONS (Questions 101 through 110): Each of the numbered items or incomplete statements in this section is followed by answers or completions of the statement. Select the ONE lettered answer or completion that is BEST in each case.

101. The F_o (fundamental frequency) is mainly responsible for pitch in cochlear implant technology. This is a frequency range from
   A. 50 to 100 Hz
   B. 100 to 200 Hz
   C. 500 to 700 Hz
   D. 1000 to 1200 Hz
   E. 2000 to 2200 Hz

102. The most prominent cells in the matrix of the spiral ligament are
   A. type I fibroblast cells
   B. type II fibroblast cells
   C. external sulcus cells
   D. intermediate cells
   E. anchoring cells

103. The nucleus multichannel cochlear implant is 25 mm long and contains approximately
   A. 5 electrodes
   B. 10 electrodes
   C. 17 electrodes
   D. 22 electrodes
   E. 27 electrodes

104. There are 13 to 16 million people in the United States with hearing loss. Of these, there are approximately how many thousand with severe to profound loss?
   A. 10,000 to 50,000
   B. 50,000 to 100,000
   C. 100,000 to 150,000
   D. 150,000 to 200,000
   E. 300,000 to 400,000

105. One notable exception to having cochlear implant is
   A. Michel deformity
   B. Mundini–Alexander deformity
   C. Alexander deformity
   D. Bing–Siebermann deformity
   E. traumatic sensorineural hearing loss

106. The current minimum age limit for implantation of a cochlear implant is age
   A. 1 year
   B. 2 years
   C. 3 years
   D. 4 years
   E. 5 years

107. A 4-year-old child has had a cochlear implant inserted in her right ear at age 3. She presents with longstanding (4 months) bilateral noninfected middle ear effusions. The next step is to
   A. suggest myringotomy with tube
   B. suggest myringotomy
   C. suggest no treatment at present and observe for infection
   D. put on high doses of antibiotics
   E. place on steroids

108. A 5-year-old female had a cochlear implant inserted successfully. The parents are told that if she has any further surgery she should avoid

   A. nitrous oxide anesthesia
   B. bipolar cautery
   C. monopolar cautery
   D. halothane anesthesia
   E. Inderal

109. Several factors are involved in predicting a more rapid or greater improvement in speech reception and production in children after cochlear implant surgery. This indicates all of the following except

   A. postlingual onset of deafness
   B. implantation during the preschool years
   C. the anatomic size of the round window
   D. a shorter period of auditory deprivation
   E. participation in an oral communication therapy program

110. The children who have been the most obvious candidates for a cochlear implant are those who have demonstrated no response to warble tones in the sound field with appropriate hearing aids or responses suggestive of vibrotactile rather than auditory sensation. This aided response is with no response above 1000 Hz but in the lower frequency having responses at levels greater than

   A. 10 to 20 dB HL
   B. 20 to 30 dB HL
   C. 30 to 40 dB HL
   D. 50 to 60 dB HL
   E. 40 to 50 dB HL

Cochlear Implants

ANSWERS AND DISCUSSION

101. (B) The F_o is 100 to 200 Hz. The first format, F_1, ranges from 200 to 1200 Hz, while F_2 ranges from 550 to 3500 Hz. (**Ref: *Essential Otolaryngology*, p. 164**)

102. (A) Type I fibroblast cells predominate. Type II fibroblast cells contain Na^+, K^+-ATPase and carbonic anhydrase ion-transporting enzymes. (**Ref: *Otolaryngology—Head and Neck Surgery*, p. 2502**)

103. (D) This is a multichannel cochlear implant and platinum rings are banded onto a tapered silastic carrier. (**Ref: *Essential Otolaryngology*, p. 164**)

104. (D) Over 90,000 of these patients may be considered candidates for cochlear implants. (**Ref: *Essential Otolaryngology*, p. 165**)

105. (A) In Michel syndrome, there is complete failure of development of the inner ear (bony and membranous aplasia). (**Ref: *Otolaryngology—Head and Neck Surgery*, p. 3144**)

106. (B) The cochlear is adult size at birth and by age 2 the mastoid antrum and facial recess, which provide access to the middle ear for active electrode placement, are adequately developed. (**Ref: *Otolaryngology—Head and Neck Surgery*, p. 3145**)

107. (C) As long as there is no infection, no treatment is necessary. **(Ref:** *Otolaryngology—Head and Neck Surgery,* **p. 3146)**

108. (C) Unipolar cautery can affect the cochlear device no matter what kind of device was inserted. **(Ref:** *Essential Otolaryngology,* **pp. 167–168)**

109. (C) The anatomic size of the round window is not a factor on the outcome of the surgery unless it is so small an implant cannot be positioned. **(Ref:** *Essential Otolaryngology,* **pp. 169–170)**

110. (E) **(Ref:** *Otolaryngology—Head and Neck Surgery,* **p. 3149)**

9

Neurotology and Skull Base Surgery

DIRECTIONS (Questons 111 through 120): Each of the numbered items or incomplete statements in this section is followed by answers or completions of the statement. Select the ONE lettered answer or completion that is BEST in each case.

111. The anterior margin of the foramen magnum is formed by the
   A. basioccipital synostosis
   B. occipital condyles
   C. hypoglossal canal
   D. parietal bone
   E. jugular foramen

112. All of the following are characteristics of neurofibroma(s) associated with Von Recklinghausen disease except
   A. multiple
   B. nonencapsulated
   C. incorporate axons
   D. malignant degeneration
   E. rapid growth

113. In performing a translabyrinthine removal of an acoustic neuroma, spinal fluid may be decompressed by opening the
   A. cochlear aqueduct
   B. vestibular aqueduct
   C. lamina cribrosa superioris
   D. lamina cribrosa posterioris
   E. sigmoid sinus

114. In performing a middle fossa procedure to remove an acoustic neuroma, generally the anterior limit of the dissection is the
   A. Bill bar
   B. cochlea
   C. facial nerve
   D. arcuate eminence
   E. middle meningeal artery

115. Transposition of the following nerve routinely occurs during a transcochlear approach
   A. V
   B. VI
   C. VII
   D. VIII
   E. X

116. The greater and lesser wings of the sphenoid bone are separated by the
   A. superior orbital fissure
   B. inferior orbital fissure
   C. foramen spinosum
   D. foramen lacerum
   E. foramen ovale

117. Identify which ganglion lies in the Meckel cave
   A. Scarpa ganglion
   B. trigeminal ganglion
   C. nodose ganglion
   D. otic ganglion
   E. olfactory ganglion

118. Anterior to the jugular foramen lies the
  A. carotid canal
  B. hypoglossal canal
  C. basioccipital synostosis
  D. internal auditory canal
  E. occipital condyles

119. For large lesions of the cerebellopontine angle, the following approach will allow the surgeon to obtain the widest field of view
  A. middle fossa
  B. translabyrinthine
  C. retrolabyrinthine
  D. suboccipital
  E. transtemporal

120. Characteristics of glomus tumors include all of the following except
  A. multicentric origin
  B. familial tendency
  C. metastatic change is rare
  D. radiation used for palliative benefit
  E. associated with neuropeptide secretion

Neurotology and Skull Base Surgery

ANSWERS AND DISCUSSION

111. (A)   The posterior skull base (posterior fossa) is bound medially by the foramen magnum, vermion fossa, and internal occipital crest and protuberance and laterally by the parietal bone. Posteriorly, it is bound by the occipital and parietal bones. **(Ref: *Essential Otolaryngology*, p. 175)**

112. (E)   Von Recklinghausen disease is an autosomal inherited disease with an incidence of 1/2500 to 1/3300 births with 50% apparent at birth. **(Ref: *Essential Otolaryngology*, pp. 1124–1125)**

113. (A)   Intracanalicular and medium-sized (2.5 cm in diameter) acoustic neuromas can be removed via the translabyrinthine approach. Larger tumors are removed via a suboccipital or retrolabyrinth approach. **(Ref: *Essential Otolaryngology*, p. 708)**

114. (E)   With removing intracanalicular acoustic neuromas that have adequate hearing preoperatively, one can preserve facial nerve function and hearing in approximately 60% of patients if surgery is approached via a middle cranial fossa approach. **(Ref: *Essential Otolaryngology* p. 708)**

115. (C) This routinely occurs in order to provide nerve access for surgery. (**Ref:** *Essential Otolaryngology,* **p. 708**)

116. (A) The superior orbital fissure lies between the roof and the lateral wall of the nose. It transmits cranial nerves III, IV, VI, V_1, the superior orbital vein, ophthalmic vein, orbital branch of the middle meningeal artery, and recurrent branch of the lacrimal artery. (**Ref:** *Essential Otolaryngology,* **p. 341**)

117. (B) The Meckel cave is a depression in the anteromedial aspect of the petrous portion of the temporal bone in which rests the gasserian ganglion of cranial nerve V. (**Ref:** *Essential Otolaryngology,* **p. 1090**)

118. (A) The jugular process, a bony ridge surrounding the posterior portion of the jugular foramen, is medial and inferior to the stylomastoid foramen. Cranial nerves IX, X, XI, and the jugular vein traverse the jugular foramen. (**Ref:** *Essential Otolaryngology,* **p. 174**)

119. (D) The main advantage of the suboccipital transmeatal approach is wide-field access to pathology and hearing preservation. Disadvantages include the upright position of the patient increases morbidity due to the possibility of air embolism, maximal cerebellar retraction is required, with potential for infarct or significant edema, and the VII nerve may not be visualized until a large portion of the tumor has been removed. (**Ref:** *Essential Otolaryngology,* **pp. 178–179**)

120. (D) With glomus jugular tumors, palliation is probably due to a reduction in vascularity, as the tumor cells are not considered to be radiosensitive. (**Ref:** *Essential Otolaryngology,* **pp. 702–703**)

10

Facial Nerve Paralysis

DIRECTIONS (Questions 121 through 140): Each of the numbered items or incomplete statements in this section is followed by answers or completions of the statement. Select the ONE lettered answer or completion that is BEST in each case.

121. A 40-year-old male presents at your office with an acute facial nerve paralysis. The differential diagnosis should include all of the following except
    A. schwannoma
    B. Lyme disease
    C. herpes zoster
    D. sarcoidosis
    E. Kawasaki disease

122. The facial nerve is not fully developed until a child is
    A. 1 year
    B. 2 years
    C. 4 years
    D. 6 years
    E. 8 years

123. The incidence of Bell's palsy per 100,000 population is
  A. 1 to 5
  B. 10 to 15
  C. 20 to 30
  D. 40 to 50
  E. 60 to 80

124. A family history of Bell's palsy is present in
  A. < 1%
  B. 2 to 3%
  C. 5%
  D. 8%
  E. 20%

125. The labyrinthine segment of the facial nerve extends from the fundus of the IAC to the facial hiatus, where the fallopian is narrowest. This segment is approximately
  A. 2 to 3 mm
  B. 3 to 5 mm
  C. 5 to 10 mm
  D. 10 to 12 mm
  E. 12 to 15 mm

126. The facial nerve has thousands of fibers. Seventy percent are myelinated and 30% sensory and secretomotor. The total number of fibers is approximately
  A. 2000
  B. 5000
  C. 10,000
  D. 20,000
  E. 25,000

127. A 60-year-old male presents to your office with a 24-hour history of right otalgia, dysgeusia, and hyperacusis. You should expect in 48 hours he may develop
  A. an otitis media
  B. a CVA
  C. Bell palsy
  D. a thrush stomatitis
  E. viral labyrinthitis

128. On testing the facial nerve in a 40-year-old male with facial nerve paralysis, there is a difference between the two sides in minimal nerve excitability testing. A difference of how many mA suggest nerve deprivation?

A. 1.0 mA
B. 3.5 mA
C. 2.0 mA
D. 2.5 mA
E. 0.5 mA

129. The incidence of severe degeneration in facial nerve paralysis with herpes zoster is approximately

A. 10%
B. 20%
C. 25%
D. 40%
E. 50%

130. Which of the following tests is used to predict facial nerve function or return 6 to 12 weeks before clinical evidence of return of function?

A. nerve excitability test
B. maximum stimulation test
C. electromyography
D. nerve conduction time
E. trigeminofacial reflex

131. A 24-year-old male presents with blistering of his right conchal bowl, facial nerve paralysis, and pain. Viral testing would show rising titers to the following virus

A. varicella–zoster
B. rhinovirus
C. herpes simplex
D. adenovirus
E. parainfluenza

132. The incidence of facial paralysis in newborns is the following
   A. 0.25% of live births
   B. 0.75% of live births
   C. 1% of live births
   D. 2% of live births
   E. 3% of live births

133. A newborn child has on examination facial diplegia, bilateral loss of abductors of the eye, extremity anomalies, and aplasia of the brachial and thoracic muscles. The most likely diagnosis is
   A. Möbius syndrome
   B. Margagni–Stewart–Morel syndrome
   C. Millard–Gubler syndrome
   D. Marie–Strümpell syndrome
   E. Myenburg syndrome

134. A large children's hospital in the midwest did a retrospective analysis of facial nerve paralysis in newborns over a 20-year period. Their study showed the following percentage of facial nerve paralysis was due to birth trauma
   A. 40%
   B. 50%
   C. 60%
   D. 70%
   E. 80%

135. A 14-year-old female was involved in an incident during which she sustained a knife wound to the central left cheek. She had a facial nerve paralysis and repair was carried out within 24 hours. She most likely had the following repair
   A. perineural repair
   B. single neurorrhaphy
   C. cable graft
   D. mastoid meatal rerouting graft
   E. epineural repair

136. A 60-year-old male presents with a peripheral facial nerve paralysis. He has a firm 2 by 3 cm parotid mass. Needle aspiration indicates a malignant tumor. The most common diagnosis is
   A. squamous cell carcinoma
   B. acinic cell carcinoma

    C. adenoid cystic carcinoma
    D. epidermal carcinoma
    E. malignant mixed carcinoma

137. The following is disruption of the nerve trunk
    A. neurotmesis
    B. axonotmesis
    C. neuropraxia
    D. synkinesia
    E. neurotrauma

138. A survey, at a large New York hospital, of temporal bone fractures revealed the following percentage of fractures involved the facial nerve
    A. 10%
    B. 20%
    C. 30%
    D. 40%
    E. 50%

139. A 30-year-old female presents to your office with recurrent orofacial edema, recurrent facial palsy, and lingua plicata (fissured tongue). The most likely diagnosis is
    A. Conradi–Hunerman syndrome
    B. Cogan syndrome
    C. Reichert syndrome
    D. Melkersson–Rosenthal syndrome
    E. Raeder syndrome

140. An 18-year-old male from Connecticut presents to your office with a facial nerve paralysis, generalized malaise, an erythematous skin lesion, regional lymphadenopathy, and a history of having camped outdoors the previous week. The most likely diagnosis is
    A. Lyme disease
    B. Kawasaki disease
    C. Chupple syndrome
    D. Bloom syndrome
    E. Bogarad syndrome

Facial Nerve Paralysis

ANSWERS AND DISCUSSION

121. (A) Schwannomas usually present as a chronic and progressive paralysis. (**Ref:** *Otolaryngology—Head and Neck Surgery,* **p. 3218**)

122. (C) The facial nerve develops and changes anatomic position until a child is 4 years old. (**Ref:** *Essential Otolaryngology,* **pp. 191–192**)

123. (C) The incidence is greater in patients over the age of 65 (60 per 100,000) and lower in children under age 13. (**Ref:** *Otolaryngology—Head and Neck Surgery,* **p. 3217**)

124. (D) Eight percent of patients with Bell's palsy will have a family history. About 0.3% of patients have bilateral paralysis and 9% have a history of previous Bell's palsy. (**Ref:** *Otolaryngology—Head and Neck Surgery,* **p. 3217**)

125. (B) This is the shortest segment. Approximately 90% of facial nerve injuries from longitudinal temporal bone fractures occur in the perigeniculate area. (**Ref:** *Essential Otolaryngology,* **p. 193**)

126. (C) The facial nerve is divided into five segments. They are the meatal, labyrinthine, tympanic, mastoid, and extratemporal segments. (**Ref:** *Essential Otolaryngology,* **pp. 193–194**)

127. (C) Initially patients with Bell's palsy may only have facial or retroauricular pain, taste disruptions, and hyperacusis. **(Ref: *Otolaryngology—Head and Neck Surgery*, p. 3218)**

128. (B) The Hilger nerve stimulator is the most common nerve excitability tester used and a difference of 3.5 mA between sides suggests nerve degeneration. **(Ref: *Otolaryngology—Head and Neck Surgery*, p. 3220)**

129. (D) With Bell's palsy, the incidence of severe degeneration is approximately 15%, whereas with herpes zoster it is 40%. **(Ref: *Essential Otolaryngology*, p. 211)**

130. (C) EMG or electromyography is not of diagnostic value until 2 weeks after degeneration as it takes 14 to 21 days after degeneration of the lower motor nerve to see spontaneous activity called fibrillation potential. Polyphasic reinnervation potentials are present 6 to 12 weeks before clinical return of facial function. **(Ref: *Essential Otolaryngology*, p. 200)**

131. (A) Ramsay–Hunt syndrome generally causes more severe symptoms and patients have a higher risk of developing complete nerve degeneration. **(Ref: *Otolaryngology—Head and Neck Surgery*, p. 3222)**

132. (A) The incidence is 0.25% of live births. The first dilemma in managing facial palsy in an infant or young child is differentiating between a true congenital paralysis and birth trauma. **(Ref: *Otolaryngology—Head and Neck Surgery*, p. 3222)**

133. (A) This is one of the common congenital syndromes that present with facial nerve paralysis. **(Ref: *Otolaryngology—Head and Neck Surgery*, p. 3225)**

134. (E) Approximately 80% of newborn facial nerve paralysis is due to birth trauma. The cases are equally divided between forceps and vaginal deliveries and cesarean sections. **(Ref: *Otolaryngology—Head and Neck Surgery*, p. 3223)**

135. **(E)** Epineural repair is preferred. Perineural repair may be applicable but only from the stylomastoid foramen to the pes anserinus. **(Ref: *Essential Otolaryngology*, p. 210)**

136. **(C)** Although adenoid cyst carcinoma incidence is only 7% of malignant tumors of the parotid gland, it has a propensity for the facial nerve. **(Ref: *Essential Otolaryngology*, pp. 207–208)**

137. **(C)** Neuropraxia is blockage of a nerve conduction due to localized pressure without axonal degeneration or nerve sheath interruption. Axonotmesis is blockage of replenishment of axoplasm to distal segment; degeneration of myelin sheath without disruption of neurolemmal sheath. **(Ref: *Essential Otolaryngology*, p. 198)**

138. **(E)** Twenty-five percent of longitudinal fractures involve the facial nerve, while 50% of transverse fractures involve the facial nerve. **(Ref: *Essential Otolaryngology*, p. 204)**

139. **(D)** In Melkersson–Rosenthal syndrome, orofacial edema is the defining feature. The complete triad is only seen in one fourth of patients. **(Ref: *Otolaryngology—Head and Neck Surgery*, p. 3226)**

140. **(A)** Lyme disease can present with facial nerve paralysis. It is caused by the tick-borne spirochete *Borrelia burgdorferi*. The primary reservoirs of the infection are the white-footed mouse and the white-tailed deer. **(Ref: *Otolaryngology—Head and Neck Surgery*, p. 3226)**

11

Syndromes and Eponyms

DIRECTIONS (Questions 141 through 155): Each of the numbered items or incomplete statements in this section is followed by answers or completions of the statement. Select the ONE lettered answer or completion that is BEST in each case.

---

141. Auriculotemporal syndrome (Frey syndrome) is associated with aberrant innervation of the sweat glands by
  A. sympathetic fibers of the VIIth cranial nerve
  B. parasympathetic fibers of the IXth cranial nerve
  C. sympathetic fibers of the IXth cranial nerve
  D. parasympathetic fibers of the VIIth cranial nerve
  E. sympathetic fibers of the Vth cranial nerve

142. A 35-year-old male presents to your office with indolent ulcers of the mucous membranes and skin with stomatitis as well as anogenital ulceration, iritis, and conjunctivitis. He has
  A. Brissaud–Marie syndrome
  B. Beckwith syndrome
  C. Bloom syndrome
  D. Alagille syndrome
  E. Behçet syndrome

143. A 45-year-old female presents to your office with a history of crocodile tears characterized by residual facial paralysis with profuse lacrimation during eating. She has
  A. Bonnier syndrome
  B. Bonnet syndrome
  C. Bogorad syndrome
  D. Besnier–Boeck–Schaumann syndrome
  E. Briquet syndrome

144. The symptom complex that occurs in individuals working in high pressures when they are returned too suddenly to normal pressure is called
  A. Caisson disease
  B. Job syndrome
  C. Hollander syndrome
  D. Tapia syndrome
  E. Still disease

145. Cavernous sinus syndrome is caused by thrombosis of the cavernous intracranial sinus and is associated with involvement of the following nerves
  A. III, IV, and V_2
  B. II, III, IV, and V_1
  C. III, IV, V_1, and V_2
  D. I, II, III, and IV
  E. III, IV, V_1, and VI

146. The syndrome of nonsyphilitic interstitial keratitis associated with vertigo, tinnitus, ataxia, and progressive sensorineural hearing loss is called
  A. Collet–Sicard syndrome
  B. Nothnagel syndrome
  C. Kallman syndrome
  D. Cogan syndrome
  E. Ortner syndrome

147. Costen syndrome is a symptom complex involving an abnormality of the
  A. temporomandibular joint
  B. retina of the eye
  C. olfactory bulb

D. posterior semicircular canal
E. petrous bone

148. DiGeorge syndrome involves cardiovascular and craniofacial anomalies and abnormalities of the
   A. trigeminal nerve
   B. olfactory bulb
   C. thyroid gland
   D. sphenopalatine ganglion
   E. thymus gland

149. The syndrome associated with leukopenia, arthritis, and enlarged lymph nodes and spleen is termed
   A. Felty syndrome
   B. Elschnig syndrome
   C. Louis–Bar syndrome
   D. Larsen syndrome
   E. Kleinschmidt's syndrome

150. A 50-year-old male presents to your office with a symptom complex of acute suppurative otitis, pain in the eye and temporal area, abducens paralysis, and diplopia. He has
   A. Dandy syndrome
   B. Gradenigo syndrome
   C. Hick syndrome
   D. Millard–Gubler syndrome
   E. Cowden syndrome

151. A 40-year-old man presents to the office with Horner syndrome. He has paralysis of the cervical sympathetic nerves and therefore has ptosis, miosis, anhidrosis, and
   A. enophalmosis
   B. exophthalmosis
   C. Frey syndrome
   D. vasomotor rhinitis
   E. diplopia

152. Vernet syndrome (jugular foramen syndrome) is associated with involvement of cranial nerves
   A. X, XI, and XII
   B. IX, X, XI, and XII
   C. IX, X, and XI
   D. X and XI
   E. XI and XII

153. Multiple endocrine adenomatosis type IIA (Sipple syndrome) is associated with hyperparathyroidism, pheochromocytoma, and
   A. pituitary adenomas
   B. medullary carcinoma of the thyroid
   C. multiple mucosal neuromas
   D. goiter
   E. an Empty–Sella phenomenon

154. Rollet syndrome is associated with involvement of cranial nerves
   A. III, IV, and V
   B. V, VI, and VII
   C. II, III, and IV
   D. III, IV, and VI
   E. IV, V, and VI

155. One of the most reliable clinical tests for hypocalcemia is the facial twitch obtained by tapping the distribution of facial nerve. This is called
   A. Chvostek sign
   B. Dupre sign
   C. Guyon sign
   D. Bryce sign
   E. Griesinger sign

Syndromes and Eponyms

ANSWERS AND DISCUSSION

141. (B) In the normal person, the sweat glands are innervated by sympathetic nerve fibers. After parotidectomy, the auriculotemporal nerve sends its parasympathetic fibers to innervate the sweat glands instead. The incidence of Frey syndrome after parotidectomy in children has been estimated to be about 20%. (**Ref:** *Essential Otolaryngology*, **p. 218**)

142. (E) The systemic manifestations of Behçet syndrome include skin, vasculature, and CNS. (**Ref:** *Otolaryngology—Head and Neck Surgery*, **p. 2934**)

143. (C) Bogorad syndrome is caused by a misdirection of regenerating autonomic fibers to the lacrimal gland instead of to the salivary gland. (**Ref:** *Essential Otolaryngology*, **p. 220**)

144. (A) Similar symptoms to Caisson disease can occur in fliers when they suddenly ascend to high altitudes unprotected by counterpressure. Symptoms include headache, pain in the epigastrium, sinuses, dyspnea, nausea, and vomiting. Nitrogen bubbles have been found in the white matter of the spinal cord. (**Ref:** *Essential Otolaryngology*, **p. 222**)

145. (B) Cavernous sinus thrombosis is a life-threatening disease that must be differentiated from orbital cellulitis. The most important clinical signs include bilateral orbital involvement, rapidly progressive severe chemosis and ophthalmoplegia, severe retinal engorgement, fever to 105°F, and prostration. The thrombosis can usually be detected on CT scanning. (**Ref:** *Otolaryngology— Head and Neck Surgery*, **p. 938**)

146. (D) In Cogan syndrome, there is visual loss and tinnitus as well. There are remissions and exacerbations. It is believed to be related to periarteritis nodosa. Treatment with steroids has been advocated. (**Ref:** *Essential Otolaryngology*, **pp. 224–225**)

147. (A) Costen syndrome is associated with the TMJ abnormality with impaired bite and is characterized by tinnitus, vertigo, and pain in the frontal, parietal, and occipital areas. (**Ref:** *Essential Otolaryngology*, **pp. 225–226**)

148. (E) There are three categories of DiGeorge syndrome. The first is a third and fourth pharyngeal pouch syndrome characterized by cardiovascular and craniofacial anomalies as well as abdominal abnormalities. The second is DiGeorge syndrome or thymus agenesis. The third is partial DiGeorge syndrome where there is thymic hypoplasia in which the thymus gland weighs less than 2 grams. (**Ref:** *Essential Otolaryngology*, **p. 227**)

149. (A) Felty syndrome is a triad of rheumatoid arthritis, splenomegaly, and neutropenia. Gastric achlorhydria is common. There is a susceptibility to infection. (**Ref:** *Essential Otolaryngology*, **p. 228**)

150. (B) Medial to the trigeminal ganglion, the abducens nerve (cranial nerve VI) passes into the cavernous sinus via the Dorello canal within the substance of the dura. Cranial nerve VI involvement within the Dorello canal is an important clinical sign for the disease of Gradenigo syndrome in cases of petrous apicitis. (**Ref:** *Otolaryngology—Head and Neck Surgery*, **p. 2485**)

151. (A) Metastatic masses, whether derived from primary tumors in the head and neck or thorax (for example, Pancoast tumor of the lung), can erode the sympathetic trunk and cause Horner syndrome. (**Ref:** *Otolaryngology—Head and Neck Surgery*, **p. 307**)

152. (C) Cranial nerve XII is spared because it is in its separate hypoglossal canal. Horner syndrome is not present because the sympathetic chain is below the foramen. This syndrome is most often caused by lymphadenopathy of the nodes of Krause in the foramen. Thrombophlebitis, tumors of the jugular bulb, and basal skull fracture can cause the syndrome. **(Ref: *Essential Otolaryngology*, p. 234)**

153. (B) MEA type II B is a variant that consists of multiple neuromas, pheochromocytoma, medullary carcinoma of the thyroid, and hyperparathyroidism. This syndrome is inherited in an autosomal dominant pattern. **(Ref: *Essential Otolaryngology*, p. 237)**

154. (D) Rollet syndrome is caused by lesions of the orbital complex. This syndrome is characterized by ptosis, diplopia, ophthalmoplegia, optic atrophy, hyperesthesia or anesthesia of the forehead, upper eyelid, and cornea, and retrobulbar neuralgia. **(Ref: *Essential Otolaryngology*, p. 224)**

155. (A) Trousseau sign is seen in hypocalcemia when a tourniquet placed around the arm causes tetany. **(Ref: *Essential Otolaryngology*, p. 254)**

12

Embryology of Clefts and Pouches

DIRECTIONS (Questions 156 through 165): Each of the numbered items or incomplete statements in this section is followed by answers or completions of the statement. Select the ONE lettered answer or completion that is BEST in each case.

156. In the embryology of the fetus, the derivatives of the five arches (pharyngeal or branchial) are of
    A. ectodermal origin
    B. a combination of ectodermal–mesodermal origin
    C. a combination of mesodermal–endodermal origin
    D. endodermal origin
    E. mesodermal origin

157. During the course of embryonic development, the third arch artery is the precursor of the
    A. arch of the aorta
    B. carotid artery
    C. subclavian artery
    D. pulmonary artery
    E. stapedial artery

158. The thymus gland is derived from
   A. the ventral aspect of the third pouch
   B. the dorsal aspect of the third pouch
   C. the ventral aspect of the fourth pouch
   D. the dorsal aspect of the fourth pouch
   E. the dorsal aspect of the second pouch

159. The second branchial arch gives rise to the
   A. IXth cranial nerve
   B. semilunar ganglion V_3
   C. geniculate ganglion VII
   D. superior laryngeal nerve
   E. recurrent laryngeal nerve

160. The cartilage bar of the fourth branchial arch forms the
   A. thyroid cartilage and cuneiform cartilage
   B. cricoid, arytenoid, and corniculate cartilage
   C. greater cornu of the hyoid
   D. upper tracheal cartilage
   E. part of the body of the hyoid

161. The ventral (thyroid) diverticulum that descends between the first and second arches can form a thyroglossal duct cyst but usually it atrophies by the
   A. fourth week of gestation
   B. fifth week of gestation
   C. sixth week of gestation
   D. seventh week of gestation
   E. eighth week of gestation

162. In the fetus, the tongue is fully developed by the
   A. fourth week
   B. sixth week
   C. eighth week
   D. 10th week
   E. 20th week

163. The hard palate is formed in the fetus by the
- **A.** fifth week
- **B.** sixth week
- **C.** seventh week
- **D.** ninth week
- **E.** 12th week

164. The incidence of esophageal artresia in cases of tracheoesophageal fistulas is slightly greater than
- **A.** 50%
- **B.** 30%
- **C.** 70%
- **D.** 60%
- **E.** 90%

165. The hyoid bone is usually calcified by age
- **A.** 4
- **B.** 10
- **C.** 20
- **D.** 2
- **E.** 8

Embryology of Clefts and Pouches

ANSWERS AND DISCUSSION

156. (E) The groove is lined by ectoderm and the pouch is lined by endoderm. Each arch has an artery, nerve, and cartilage bar. The nerves are anterior to their respective arteries except in the fifth arch where the nerve is posterior to the artery. (**Ref:** *Essential Otolaryngology*, **pp. 259–260**)

157. (B) During the course of embryonic development, the first and second arch arteries degenerate. The second arch artery has an upper branch that passes through a mass of mesoderm, which later chondrifies and ossifies as the stapes. (**Ref:** *Essential Otolaryngology*, **p. 260**)

158. (A) The dorsal aspect of the second pouch and the dorsal aspect of the third pouch form the parathyroid glands. (**Ref:** *Essential Otolaryngology*, **p. 263**)

159. (C) The first branchial arch gives rise to the semilunar ganglion V_3 and the third arch gives rise to the IXth cranial nerve. The fourth arch gives rise to the superior laryngeal nerve and the fifth arch gives rise to the recurrent laryngeal nerve. (**Ref:** *Essential Otolaryngology*, **p. 262**)

160. (A) The cartilage bar of the fourth arch forms the thyroid cartilage, and can form cartilage, while the cartilage bar of the fifth arch forms the cricoid, arytenoid, and corniculate. **(Ref:** *Essential Otolaryngology,* **p. 266)**

161. (C) The ventral diverticulum is situated between the tuberculum impar and the copula. The tuberculum impar together with the lingual swellings become the anterior two thirds of the tongue, and the copula is the precursor of the posterior of the tongue. **(Ref:** *Essential Otolaryngology,* **pp. 266–267)**

162. (E) The tongue is derived from ectodermal origin (anterior two thirds) and entodermal origin (posteriorly). At the seventh week, the somites from the high cervical area differentiate into voluntary muscle of the tongue. The circumvallate papillae develop between the 8th and the 20th weeks. **(Ref:** *Essential Otolaryngology,* **p. 267)**

163. (D) The soft palate and the uvula are completed by the 11th to 12th week. From the 8th week to the 24th week of embryonic life, the nostrils are occupied by an epithelial plug. Failure to resorb this epithelium results in atresia or stenosis of the anterior nares. **(Ref:** *Essential Otolaryngology,* **p. 269)**

164. (E) During embryonic development, when a single tubal structure is to later become two tubal structures, the original tube is first obliterated by a proliferation of lining epithelium, then, as resorption of the epithelium takes place, the second tube is formed and the first tube is recannulized. Hence any malformation usually involves both tubes. **(Ref:** *Essential Otolaryngology,* **p. 270)**

165. (D) The thyroid cartilage starts to calcify at age 20 from the inferior margin and the superior margin never calcifies. The hyoid bone calcifies by age 2. **(Ref:** *Essential Otolaryngology,* **p. 272)**

13

Cleft Lip and Palate

DIRECTIONS (Questions 166 through 180): Each of the numbered
items or incomplete statements in this section is followed by answers or
completions of the statement. Select the ONE lettered answer or completion that is BEST in each case.

---

166. The muscle that is the primary elevator of the soft palate is the
  - **A.** tensor veli palatini
  - **B.** levator veli palatini
  - **C.** musculus uvulae
  - **D.** glossopalatine
  - **E.** palatopharyngeus

167. An incomplete cleft lip involves a portion of the lip and may form
a muscular diastasis with intact underlying skin to a large cleft
with only a small band of residual tissue connecting the two sides
of the lip. This band is called the
  - **A.** tubercle
  - **B.** philtrum
  - **C.** Cupid bow
  - **D.** Simonart bar
  - **E.** vermilion band

168. The embryologic development of the lip and palate occurs between
- **A.** 2 and 5 weeks
- **B.** 4 and 7 weeks
- **C.** 8 and 10 weeks
- **D.** 10 and 13 weeks
- **E.** 13 and 16 weeks

169. A neworn child is noted to have an incomplete cleft of the palate. This probably occurred at the following point in embryologic development
- **A.** 2 to 5 weeks
- **B.** 4 to 7 weeks
- **C.** 7 to 12 weeks
- **D.** 12 to 14 weeks
- **E.** 14 to 18 weeks

170. In your office, you have a mother who had a cleft palate repaired as a child. She has one child without congenital deformities but she is 12 weeks pregnant. You can advise her that the chance of this child having a cleft palate alone is
- **A.** 2%
- **B.** 6%
- **C.** 15%
- **D.** 25%
- **E.** 50%

171. The incidence of a cleft deformity per live births is
- **A.** 1:200
- **B.** 1:550
- **C.** 1:680
- **D.** 1:1000
- **E.** 1:2020

172. A child is seen in the neonatal nursery with a cleft palate deformity. The parents are very anxious to have this repaired. You suggest they should wait until
- **A.** 2 to 3 months
- **B.** 5 to 6 months
- **C.** 10 to 12 months

D. 16 to 18 months
E. 18 to 24 months

173. You are asked to see a child in the newborn nursery with a cleft lip deformity only. The parents want an idea of when this can be surgically repaired. You tell the parents this can usually be done at
A. 4 weeks
B. 6 weeks
C. 8 weeks
D. 10 weeks
E. 14 weeks

174. Lip adhesion is a preliminary procedure used in the therapy of cleft lip repair. In the procedure, there are usually laterally based flaps obtained from the lip itself. The procedure is usually done at
A. 1 to 4 weeks
B. 4 to 8 weeks
C. 8 to 12 weeks
D. 12 to 16 weeks
E. 16 to 20 weeks

175. One of the palatoplasties done for a soft palate deformity using posteriorly and anteriorly based unipedicle microperiosteal flaps is called a(n)
A. Oxford procedure
B. Von Langenbeck procedure
C. Millard procedure
D. Schweckendick procedure
E. Smith procedure

176. The procedure used to close the soft palate cleft with closure of the hard palate at a later date is called a(n)
A. Von Langenbeck procedure
B. Schweckendick procedure
C. Oxford procedure
D. Millard procedure
E. Smith procedure

177. The most common complication of palatoplasty procedures is
    A. fistula formation
    B. necrosis of flap
    C. hypernasal speech
    D. dysphagia
    E. hemorrhage

178. The Dibbell technique is a procedure to correct the
    A. soft palate
    B. hard palate
    C. lip only
    D. lip and hard palate
    E. nasal and lip

179. The technique used to lengthen the columella in cleft lip repair is the
    A. Dibbell
    B. Millard
    C. Bardach
    D. Von Langenbeck
    E. Smith

180. The primary complication of a pharyngeal flap initially is
    A. infection
    B. necrosis
    C. hemorrhage
    D. fistula
    E. pain

Cleft Lip and Palate

ANSWERS AND DISCUSSION

166. (B) The levator veli palatini elevates the palate. The tensor veli palatini tenses and depresses the soft palate, while the musculus uvulae drains the uvula upward and forward. Both the glossopalatine and the palatopharyngeus draw the palate down and narrow the pharynx. (**Ref:** *Essential Otolaryngology,* **p. 278**)

167. (D) This band of tissue is the Simonart bar. (**Ref:** *Otolaryngology—Head and Neck Surgery,* **p. 1128**)

168. (B) The lip and primary palate develop early at 4 to 7 weeks. Clefts of this area probably result from a failure of a mesodermal delivery or proliferation from the midline frontonasal process and lateral maxillary process. (**Ref:** *Otolaryngology—Head and Neck Surgery,* **pp. 1129–1131**)

169. (C) The secondary palate develops at 7 to 12 weeks. It is formed by medial growths of the palatal shelves of the maxilla, which eventually fuse together during normal development. (**Ref:** *Otolaryngology—Head and Neck Surgery,* **p. 1131**)

170. (B) There would be a 6% chance of having a cleft palate and a 4% chance of having a cleft lip with or without a cleft palate. (**Ref:** *Essential Otolaryngology,* **p. 280**)

171. **(C)** A cleft deformity occurs approximately in 1 of every 680 births. In general, 10 to 30% are isolated cleft lips, 35 to 55% involve both the primary and secondary palate (cleft lip and palate), and 30 to 45% involve only the secondary palate. (**Ref:** *Otolaryngology—Head and Neck Surgery,* **p. 1132**)

172. **(E)** Most experts perform cleft lip repair during the third month of life and cleft palate repair following eruption of the first molars, at approximately age 18 to 24 months. (**Ref:** *Essential Otolaryngology,* **p. 281**)

173. **(D)** In the United States, the rule of 10s exists. With a cleft lip you want to wait until a child is at least 10 weeks old, weighs 10 pounds, and has a hemoglobin of 10 grams. (**Ref:** *Otolaryngology—Head and Neck Surgery,* **p. 1137**)

174. **(A)** Lip adhesion is usually performed in the first month of life with a definitive lip repair done at age 4 to 7 months. (**Ref:** *Otolaryngology—Head and Neck Surgery,* **p. 1138**)

175. **(A)** This is called the Oxford palatoplasty. The advantages of this is that it lengthens the palate and patients usually have better speech than they would have with Von Langenbeck palatoplasty. (**Ref:** *Otolaryngology—Head and Neck Surgery,* **p. 1146**)

176. **(B)** The advantages of this procedure include the construction of a velopharyngeal valve at an early age, minimal disturbance in future facial growth, and the frequent occurrence of significant narrowing of the width of the remaining palatal cleft with increasing age. (**Ref:** *Otolaryngology—Head and Neck Surgery,* **p. 1147**)

177. **(C)** The most common complication of palatoplasty is hypernasal speech, which may occur in up to 30% of cleft palate patients. Fistula formation is from 10 to 21%. (**Ref:** *Otolaryngology—Head and Neck Surgery,* **p. 1151**)

178. **(E)** The Dibbell technique is used for the nasal ala, the lateral alar margin, and the lip. (**Ref:** *Otolaryngology—Head and Neck Surgery,* **p. 1153**)

179. (C) The Bardach technique is a method of correction to lengthen the columella by the use of a triangular skin flap from the middle portion of the upper lip in both unilateral and bilateral cleft nasal deformities. (**Ref:** *Otolaryngology—Head and Neck Surgery*, **p. 1154**)

180. (C) Hemorrhage is the most frequent initial complication of a pharyngeal flap as it will usually occur in the first 24 hours. Control must be obtained and good airway preserved. (**Ref:** *Otolaryngology—Head and Neck Surgery*, **p. 1160**)

14

Immunology and Allergy

DIRECTIONS (Questions 181 through 190): Each of the numbered items or incomplete statements in this section is followed by answers or completions of the statement. Select the ONE lettered answer or completion that is BEST in each case.

---

181. Identify which statement is incorrect.
    A. Pollen comes from the anther of the stamen.
    B. Anemophilous means water soluble.
    C. Fungi do not contain chlorophyll.
    D. Mite is the most important antigen in dust.
    E. Allergic contact dermatitis is a type IV cell-mediated delayed hypersensitivity.

182. The third most abundant serum immunoglobulin that inhibits the adherence of microorganisms and alien macromolecules is
    A. IgA
    B. IgD
    C. IgE
    D. IgG
    E. IgM

183. Tests of B-cell function include all of the following except
    A. measurement of serum levels of immunoglobulins
    B. antibody response following immunization

C. PRIST
D. tests of lymphokine production
E. presence of plasma cells

184. The principle organs that serve as sites for proliferation and development of cells involved in immune responses include all the following except
   A. bone marrow
   B. Peyer patches of the gastrointestinal tract
   C. liver
   D. lymph nodes
   E. spleen

185. Identify which statement is correct.
   A. IgE antibodies attach to membranes of eosinophils, as many as 80,000 molecules per cell.
   B. Toxic–complex reactions occur when IgM antibodies combine with fixed antigen.
   C. Cellular hypersensitivity occurs 24 to 72 hours after antigen introduction.
   D. Reagin is a heat-stable transferable skin sensitizing factor.
   E. IgA and reagin are the same.

186. Tests of T-cell function include all of the following except
   A. lymphocyte count and morphology
   B. E-rosette assay
   C. allogenic skin graft rejection
   D. delayed hypersensitivity skin tests
   E. nitroblue trazolium test

187. Identify which statement is incorrect.
   A. Phenylephrine is an alpha-adrenergic agent.
   B. Epinephrine has alpha and beta activity.
   C. Immunotherapy is effective when appropriately applied to those with known atopic IgE-mediated disease.
   D. With appropriate immune therapy, there is a documented increase of IgG-blocking antibody in the serum.
   E. Corticosteroids affect the sodium pump, reduce capillary permeability, and stabilize lysosomal membranes.

188. What am I? I belong to a family of 20 carbon unsaturated hydroxyaliphatic. My synthesis can be inhibited by nonsteroidal antiinflammatory agents.
   A. leukotrienes
   B. eosinophol chemotactic factor
   C. histamine
   D. prostaglandins
   E. complement

189. Identify which statement is incorrect.
   A. With chemotaxis, there is a random movement of cells.
   B. The in vivo test for chemotaxis is the Rebuck Skin Window.
   C. The nitroblue trazolium test is a screening test for phagocytosis.
   D. Opsonins interfere with microorganisms to aid their digestion by phagocytic cells.
   E. IgE and complement C3b are opsonins.

190. The following percentage of the United States population suffers from allergic disease
   A. < 5%
   B. 5 to 10%
   C. 15 to 20%
   D. 25 to 30%
   E. > 30%

Immunology and Allergy

ANSWERS AND DISCUSSION

181. (B) Type I is an IgE-mediated reaction via mast cells, type II is a cytotoxic reaction, type III is an immune complex-mediated reaction, and type IV is a cell-mediated reaction. **(Ref: *Essential Otolaryngology*, pp. 300–301)**

182. (A) IgG is the major antibody of secondary responses, IgM is the predominant antibody in early immune response, IgD is found in large quantities in circulatory B cells, and IgE is found in basophils and mast cells. IgA is the predominant Ig in seromucous secretions. **(Ref: *Essential Otolaryngology*, p. 299)**

183. (D) About 10 to 15% of lymphocytes have surface IgG and are designated as B cells. These cells have been designated as B cells in mammals in recognition of the bursa of Fabricus. **(Ref: *Otolaryngology—Head and Neck Surgery*, p. 258)**

184. (C) The primary lymphoid system includes the major sites of lymphopoiesis (the thymus and bone marrow) and the secondary lymphoid system provides the environment that enhances antigen–effector cell interactions (Walder Ring, lymph nodes, spleen, and Peyer patches). **(Ref: *Essential Otolaryngology*, pp. 297–298)**

185. (C) Type IV reaction is a cell-mediated delayed hypersensitivity reaction. **(Ref: *Essential Otolaryngology*, pp. 301–302)**

186. (E) T cells are important for many reasons. One of their dramatic features is their early recognition of foreign antigens present on the surface of accessory cells such as macrophages, dendritic cells, and Langerhans cells. (**Ref:** *Otolaryngology—Head and Neck Surgery,* **pp. 259–260)**

187. (A) Phenylephrine is an alpha-adrenergic agent but is a vasoconstrictor. Phenylephrine is used mainly as a nasal decongestant, a pressor agent in hypotension, a mydriatic, and a local vasoconstrictor. (**Ref:** *Essential Otolaryngology,* **p. 309)**

188. (D) Prostaglandins are produced by nearly all body tissues. They are potent vasodilators, regulate platelet aggregation, and promote diuresis. (**Ref:** *Essential Otolaryngology,* **p. 295)**

189. (A) In chemotaxis, there is a very organized movement of cells. (**Ref:** *Essential Otolaryngology,* **p. 293)**

190. (C) An allergen is an antigen that causes allergic reaction. An allergic reaction is an immune response with a deleterious effect on the host. Allergic reactions are divided by the Gell and Coombs classification into four types. The first three are mediated by antibody, the fourth by T cells and macrophages. (**Ref:** *Essential Otolaryngology,* **p. 300)**

15

The Chest

191. The volume of gas that is either inspired or expired during each normal respiratory cycle is called the
   A. tidal volume
   B. residual volume
   C. total lung capacity
   D. functional residual capacity
   E. forced expiratory volume (FEV)

192. One of the most useful tests for asthmatics to monitor the severity of an asthmatic attack is
   A. total lung capacity
   B. vital capacity
   C. forced expiratory volume
   D. tidal volume
   E. residual volume

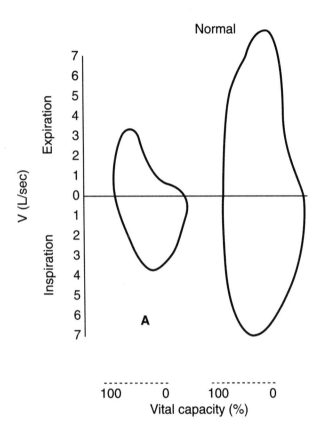

193. The above low volume loop labeled A is indicative of
    A. pulmonary emphysema
    B. asthma
    C. pulmonary fibrosis
    D. chronic obstructive pulmonary disease (COPD)
    E. chronic bronchitis

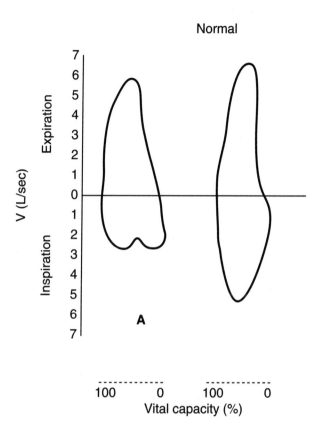

194. The above flow loop A is indicative of
    A. COPD
    B. pulmonary fibrosis
    C. pulmonary emphysema
    D. asthma
    E. extrathoracic obstruction

195. A measure of the distensibility of the lung parenchyma is called
    A. functional residual capacity
    B. diffusing capacity
    C. compliance
    D. tidal volume
    E. FEV$_1$

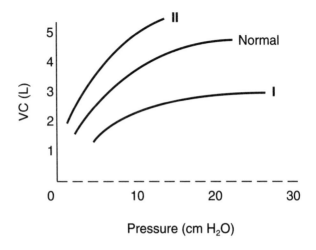

196. Line I is indicative of
    A. emphysema
    B. COPD
    C. pulmonary fibrosis
    D. asthma
    E. chronic bronchitis

197. Normal lung function is considered to have an alveolar–arterial (A–a) gradient of less than
    A. 20 mm Hg
    B. 25 mm Hg
    C. 30 mm Hg
    D. 35 mm Hg
    E. 40 mm Hg

198. FEV_1 should be the following percentage or greater of the predicted volume from a normative chart
    A. 40%
    B. 50%
    C. 60%
    D. 70%
    E. 80%

199. Total lung capacity for males is
  A. 3 liters
  B. 4 liters
  C. 5 liters
  D. 6 liters
  E. 7 liters

200. A class I congenital agenesis of the lung has been classified by Schneider as
  A. only trachea present
  B. no pulmonary tissue present with a normal trachea
  C. no pulmonary tissue present with a normal bronchi
  D. total agenesis
  E. normal pulmonary tissue and no trachea or bronchi

201. A methemoglobin level of this degree produces cynanosis.
  A. 70.5 mg/dL
  B. 71 mg/dL
  C. 72 mg/dL
  D. 73 mg/dL
  E. 75 mg/dL

202. The leading primary pulmonary carcinoma in women is
  A. oat cell carcinoma
  B. squamous cell carcinoma
  C. adenocarcinoma
  D. adenoid cystic carcinoma
  E. mucoepidermoid carcinoma

203. The triad of an apical lung tumor, vocal cord paralysis, and Horner syndrome is called
  A. Bourneville syndrome
  B. Bonnier syndrome
  C. Pancoast syndrome
  D. Forney syndrome
  E. Dalange syndrome

204. The thyroidea ima artery is present in the following percentage of the population
  A. 5%
  B. 10%
  C. 20%
  D. 30%
  E. 40%

205. The following percentage of mediastinal tumors are malignant
  A. 5%
  B. 10%
  C. 20%
  D. 30%
  E. 40%

206. A 6-month-old child is taken to the operating room to have a peanut removed from her right main stem bronchus. The size of the bronchoscope you would most likely choose would be
  A. 2.0 mm
  B. 3.0 mm
  C. 3.5 mm
  D. 4.5 mm
  E. 6.0 mm

207. In the adult male, the average distance from the incisor teeth to the hiatus is
  A. 28 cm
  B. 38 cm
  C. 44 cm
  D. 50 cm
  E. 55 cm

208. The most common cause of hemoptysis related to the lung is
  A. mitral stenosis
  B. tuberculosis
  C. tracheobronchitis
  D. bronchiectasis
  E. adenoma

209. The most common cause of dysphagia lusoria is an abnormal
   - **A.** subclavian artery
   - **B.** innominate artery
   - **C.** pulmonary artery
   - **D.** aorta
   - **E.** carotid artery

210. The ligamentum arteriosus is an abnormality of the following branchial arch
   - **A.** first
   - **B.** second
   - **C.** third
   - **D.** fourth
   - **E.** fifth

The Chest

ANSWERS AND DISCUSSION

191. (A) The residual volume is the amount of gas that remains in the lungs at the end of a maximal expiratory effort. (**Ref:** *Essential Otolaryngology*, **p. 319**)

192. (C) The forced expiratory volume is one of the best measures to monitor an asthmatic attack at home. This is the volume of gas exhaled from the lung after initiation of a forceful exhalation following a maximal inspiration. (**Ref:** *Essential Otolaryngology*, **p. 319**)

193. (D) This flow volume curve is indicative of COPD. The flow volume curves also allow the pulmonologist to evaluate the upper airway. (**Ref:** *Essential Otolaryngology*, **pp. 320–321**)

194. (E) This is indicative of extrathoracic obstruction or upper airway obstruction. (**Ref:** *Essential Otolaryngology*, **pp. 321–322**)

195. (C) The compliance of the lung refers to the elastic properties of that organ. (**Ref:** *Essential Otolaryngology*, **pp. 322–323**)

196. (C) This is indicative of pulmonary fibrosis. Line II is indicative of pulmonary emphysema. (**Ref:** *Essential Otolaryngology*, **pp. 322–323**)

197. (A) If there is less than a 20 mm Hg gradient between the alveolar and arterial oxygen tensions, it is likely that the lungs are normal and that alveolar hypoventilation is the sole abnormality producing the hypoxemia. (**Ref:** *Essential Otolaryngology,* **p. 324**)

198. (E) FEV_1 should be 80% or greater of predicted values and it is important in measuring asthma severity. (**Ref:** *Essential Otolaryngology,* **p. 326**)

199. (D) For males, the total lung capacity is 6 liters and for females is 4.2 liters. (**Ref:** *Essential Otolaryngology,* **p. 326**)

200. (D) Class I congenital agenesis is total agenesis of the lung as classified by Schneider. In Class II, only the trachea is present and in Class III the trachea and bronchi are present without any pulmonary tissue. (**Ref:** *Essential Otolaryngology,* **p. 327**)

201. (E) Hypoxemia is defined as less than 75% oxygen saturation or less than 40 mm Hg PO_2. (**Ref:** *Essential Otolaryngology,* **pp. 327–328**)

202. (C) In females, squamous cell carcinoma is the leading primary pulmonary carcinoma. (**Ref:** *Essential Otolaryngology,* **p. 327**)

203. (C) This is Pancoast syndrome and presents with shoulder pain, hand atrophy, and Horner syndrome. (**Ref:** *Essential Otolaryngology,* **p. 327**)

204. (B) Ten percent of the population has a thyroidea ima artery. It arises from either the innominate artery or the aorta and passes upward along the anterior aspect of the trachea. (**Ref:** *Essential Otolaryngology,* **p. 329**)

205. (D) Approximately 30 to 33% are malignant. The most common is lymphoma. (**Ref:** *Essential Otolaryngology,* **p. 334**)

206. (C) A 3.5-mm bronchoscope would be an appropriate size. (**Ref:** *Essential Otolaryngology,* **p. 335**)

207. (B) In a 3-year-old, this would be approximately 23 cm. **(Ref:** *Essential Otolaryngology,* **p. 335)**

208. (D) Bronchiectasis is the most common cause of hemoptysis. **(Ref:** *Essential Otolaryngology,* **p. 336)**

209. (A) An abnormal subclavian artery arising from the descending aorta is the most common cause of dysphagia lusoria (dysphagia caused by an aberrant great vessel). **(Ref:** *Essential Otolaryngology,* **p. 337)**

210. (D) Ligamentum arteriosus is due to the persistence of the right fourth branchial arch vessel becoming the aorta instead of the left fourth arch vessel. This vessel crosses the trachea causing an anterior compression. **(Ref:** *Essential Otolaryngology,* **pp. 336–337)**

16

Related Ophthalmology

Each of the numbered items or incomplete statements in this section is followed by answers or completions of the statement. Select the ONE lettered answer or completion that is BEST in each case.

211. The floor of the orbit is formed by the orbital plate of the maxilla, orbital surface of the zygoma, and the
    A. lacrimal bone
    B. sphenoid bone
    C. orbital process of palatine bone
    D. orbital process of the frontal bone
    E. lesser wing of the sphenoid

212. A 20-year-old male sustained eye trauma and it was determined he had a displaced trochlea. The physical exam would have revealed
    A. diplopia on downward gaze
    B. diplopia on lateral gaze
    C. diplopia on upward gaze
    D. enophthalmos
    E. diplopia on medial gaze

213. A 35-year-old male presents to your office with proptosis, excessive lacrimation, periorbital edema, and photophobia. One test that would be helpful in making a diagnosis would be a
   A. TSH assay
   B. CBC
   C. ESR
   D. SGOT and SGPT
   E. urinalysis

214. The leading cause of adult onset unilateral exophthalmus is
   A. Graves disease
   B. mucocele
   C. lymphoma
   D. intraorbital hemangioma
   E. lymphangioma

215. The superior orbital fissure transmits the superior orbital vein, ophthalmic vein, orbital branch of the middle meningeal artery, the recurrent branch of the lacrimal artery, and cranial nerves
   A. III, V_1
   B. III, V_1, V_2
   C. III, IV, V_1
   D. III, IV, VI, V_1
   E. III, IV, VI

216. The usual causative organism in cavernous sinus thrombosis is
   A. coagulase-positive *S. aureus*
   B. *H. influenzae*
   C. *Strep. pyogenes*
   D. *Strep. pneumoniae*
   E. *Moraxella catarrhalis*

217. The orbital decompression procedure in which the floor and the medial wall of the orbit are removed to allow expansion into the ethmoid and maxillary sinuses was first described by
   A. Ogura
   B. Kronlein
   C. Sewell
   D. Hirsch
   E. Naffziger

218. The lateral rectus muscle is innervated by the following cranial nerve
    A. IIIrd nerve
    B. IInd nerve
    C. IVth nerve
    D. VIth nerve
    E. V₁th nerve

219. The muscles involved with movement of the eyes down and to the right are the
    A. right lateral rectus and left medial rectus
    B. right medial rectus and left lateral rectus
    C. right superior rectus and left inferior oblique
    D. right inferior oblique and left superior rectus
    E. right inferior rectus and left superior oblique

220. The procedure for decompression for malignant exophthalmus in which an ethmoidectomy is done and the floor of the frontal sinus is removed is described by
    A. Kronlein
    B. Sewell
    C. Naffziger
    D. Hirsch
    E. Ogura

Related Ophthalmology

ANSWERS AND DISCUSSION

211. **(C)** The orbit is a quadrilateral pyramid with a floor, roof, medial wall, and a lateral wall. (**Ref:** *Essential Otolaryngology,* **p. 341**)

212. **(A)** The trochlea is a pulley through which runs the tendon of the superior oblique muscle and it is located between the roof and the medial wall. Disruption causes diplopia on downward gaze. (**Ref:** *Essential Otolaryngology,* **p. 341**)

213. **(A)** One would suspect Graves disease and therefore a TSH assay is the most sensitive test for recognition of subtle degrees of hyperthyroidism. Ten percent of Graves patients have no demonstrable thyroid disease. (**Ref:** *Otolaryngology—Head and Neck Surgery,* **p. 2473**)

214. **(A)** Diseases that can mimic bilateral Graves ophthalmopathy include Wegener granulomatosis, inflammatory pseudotumor, and cavernous sinus thrombosis. (**Ref:** *Otolaryngology—Head and Neck Surgery,* **p. 2473**)

215. **(D)** The superior orbital fissure lies between the roof and the lateral wall of the nose. It is a gap between the lesser and the greater wings of the sphenoid. (**Ref:** *Essential Otolaryngology,* **p. 341**)

216. (A) Coagulase-positive *S. aureus* is the most common organism in cavernous sinus thrombosis. (**Ref:** *Essential Otolaryngology,* p. 747)

217. (A) In the Ogura procedure, one does as complete an ethmoidectomy as possible and one also decompresses the floor of the orbit. (**Ref:** *Otolaryngology—Head and Neck Surgery,* p. 2474)

218. (D) A good formula for remembering this is LR_6 (SO_4), the rest by III. The lateral rectus is innervated by the VIth cranial nerve and the superior oblique by the IVth cranial nerve. The remainder is by the IIIrd cranial nerve. (**Ref:** *Essential Otolaryngology,* p. 343)

219. (E) (**Ref:** *Essential Otolaryngology,* p. 343)

220. (B) In the Sewell procedure, an ethmoidectomy is performed and the floor of the frontal sinus is removed. In the Kronlein procedure, the lateral orbital wall is removed, and in the Hirsch procedure, the orbital floor is removed. (**Ref:** *Essential Otolaryngology,* p. 344)

17

Related Neurology

DIRECTIONS (Questions 221 through 235): Each of the numbered items or incomplete statements in this section is followed by answers or completions of the statement. Select the ONE lettered answer or completion that is BEST in each case.

221. Internuclear ophthalmoplegia is pathognomic of
    A. myasthenia gravis
    B. vascular migraine
    C. temporal arteritus
    D. multiple sclerosis
    E. Guillian–Barré

222. The Charcot triad in multiple sclerosis includes nystagmus, scanning speech, and
    A. diplopia
    B. urinary retention
    C. muscle retention
    D. dysphagia
    E. intention tremor

223. A 40-year-old female presents to your office with papilledema, headache, vomiting, and a giant imbalance. She has also paraxysmal positional nystagmus in all directions. An MRI scan is most likely to reveal a
    A. cerebellar glioma
    B. meningioma
    C. Chiari malformation
    D. CVA
    E. normal exam

224. A 65-year-old male is seen on consultation in the hospital with spontaneous nystagmus, ipsilateral Horner syndrome, ipsilateral loss of pain and temperature sensation, and ipsilateral rectus muscle and facial weakness. He has
    A. lateral pontomedullary syndrome
    B. cerebellar infarction
    C. Friedreich ataxia
    D. Wallenberg syndrome
    E. multiple sclerosis

225. A 75-year-old male, with a history of ASHD, presents to your office with a history of recurrent vertigo that lasts for several minutes and is associated with nausea and vomiting. He also gets visual illusions and hallucinations, drop attacks, visual field defects, and diplopia. The most likely diagnosis is
    A. benign paroxysmal vertigo
    B. vertebrobasilar insufficiency
    C. cerebellar infarction
    D. meningioma
    E. migraine

226. A mother brings to you her 8-month-old child who periodically gets episodes of head tilt, pallor, vomiting, and agitation. The episodes of head tilt can last from a few hours to 3 days. You make the diagnosis of paroxysmal torticollis. The treatment is
    A. none
    B. muscle relaxants
    C. antibiotic therapy
    D. low dose Inderol
    E. physiotherapy

227. A 12-year-old boy is brought into your office by his parents. He has a history of periodic episodes of difficulty swallowing and diplopia. He also notices that he gets weak after exercise and at the end of the day. After examination, the next step is to order a
   A. tensilon test
   B. CT scan of head
   C. Ba swallow
   D. exercise cardiogram
   E. psychologic assessment

228. A 45-year-old farmer presents to your office with a history of fever, parotid swelling, uveitis, and transient bilateral facial nerve paralysis. The most likely diagnosis is
   A. pituitary adenoma
   B. temporal arteritis
   C. uveoparotid fever of Heerfordt
   D. myasthenia gravis
   E. relapsing polychondritis

229. A 45-year-old female presents to your office with a history of headache and visual symptoms. On examination, you discover the patient has bitemporal hemianopsia. The most likely diagnosis is
   A. pituitary adenoma
   B. cavernous sinus syndrome
   C. craniopharyngioma
   D. cerebellar tumor
   E. meningioma

230. A 40-year-old male has undergone surgery 18 hours previously for a pituitary adenoma. The nurse phones and says that his urinary output is greater than 250 mL/hr with a specific gravity of 1.0. Your initial treatment would be intravenous fluids and
   A. DDAVP
   B. Inderol
   C. cortisone acetate
   D. demedocycline
   E. bumex

231. A sense of foul smell when none is present is called
   A. parosmia
   B. hyperosmia

   C. hyposmia
   D. anosmia
   E. cacosmia

232. The following medication has been used in the treatment of anosmia
   A. Tegretol
   B. Inderol
   C. Dilantin
   D. vitamin A
   E. Inderol

233. Friedreich ataxia is an autosomal recessive disorder in which patients lose their ability to ambulate independently 10 to 20 years after onset. The most life-threatening aspects of the disease are related to
   A. neurologic manifestations
   B. cardiac manifestations
   C. renal manifestations
   D. pulmonary manifestations
   E. gastrointestinal manifestations

234. Refsum syndrome is a familial disorder that is believed to be inherited in an autosomal recessive fashion. Patients have retinitis pigmentosa, cerebral ataxia, and sensorineural hearing loss. Serum analysis would reveal elevated
   A. ESR
   B. SGOT, SGPT
   C. creatinine
   D. phytanic acid
   E. PT, PTT

235. The second most common cerebral pontine angle mass lesion is a
   A. glioma
   B. aneurysm
   C. epidermoid
   D. metastatic neoplasma
   E. meningioma

Related Neurology

ANSWERS AND DISCUSSION

221. (D) With internuclear ophthalmoplegia, the internal rectus on one side is paralyzed and the external rectus on the opposite side is weak, thus producing nystagmoid jerks of the outwardly deviating eye. (**Ref:** *Essential Otolaryngology*, **p. 345**)

222. (E) Multiple sclerosis has an inherited predisposition, although it is not inherited according to Mendelian laws. (**Ref:** *Essential Otolaryngology*, **p. 345**)

223. (A) There is an incidence of papilledema in 90% of patients with a cerebral glioma. (**Ref:** *Otolaryngology—Head and Neck Surgery*, **p. 3188**)

224. (D) The zone of infarction producing the lateral medullary syndrome consists of a wedge of the dorsolateral medulla just posterior to the olive. (**Ref:** *Otolaryngology—Head and Neck Surgery*, **p. 3185**)

225. (B) Vertebrobasilar insufficiency is a common cause of vertigo in the elderly. (**Ref:** *Otolaryngology—Head and Neck Surgery*, **pp. 3183–3184**)

226. (A) No treatment is necessary with paroxysmal torticollis and in most children the spells stop spontaneously by age 5. (**Ref:** *Otolaryngology—Head and Neck Surgery*, **p. 3183**)

227. (A)   More than likely the child has myasthenia gravis and a tensilon test will be positive. (Ref: *Essential Otolaryngology,* pp. 346–347)

228. (C)   Uveoparotid fever of Heerfordt is a variant of sarcoidosis. (Ref: *Essential Otolaryngology,* p. 348)

229. (A)   This is the classic presentation of a pituitary adenoma. (Ref: *Essential Otolaryngology,* pp. 351–352)

230. (A)   The patient has diabetes insipidus and treatment is intravenous fluids at a rate to replace the previous hours' output and desmopressin acetate (DDAVP), a synthetic analog of vasopressin. (Ref: *Essential Otolaryngology,* pp. 353–354)

231. (E)   Cacosmia is a sense of foul smell when none is present. In anosmia, ammonia stimulates cranial nerve V and not cranial nerve I. Hence, it can be used as a diagnostic test when a psychogenic cause of anosmia is suspected. (Ref: *Essential Otolaryngology,* p. 356)

232. (D)   Vitamin A has been used in the past for anosmia with mixed results. (Ref: *Essential Otolaryngology,* p. 356)

233. (B)   The mean age of onset of Friedreich ataxia is between ages 8 and 13. The ataxia is progressive. (Ref: *Otolaryngology—Head and Neck Surgery,* p. 3193)

234. (D)   Elevated phytanic acid provides a diagnostic test for Refsum syndrome. Reduction of this by dietary control is an important aspect in treatment. (Ref: *Otolaryngology—Head and Neck Surgery,* p. 3195)

235. (E)   Meningiomas usually present with headaches and multiple nerve palsies. With large ones, brainstem and cerebellar signs may be present. (Ref: *Essential Otolaryngology,* p. 355)

18

Fluids, Electrolytes, and Acid–Base Balance

DIRECTIONS (Questions 236 through 245): Each of the numbered items or incomplete statements in this section is followed by answers or completions of the statement. Select the ONE lettered answer or completion that is BEST in each case.

---

236. The average 70-kg man contains the following amount of intracellular fluid
   A. 20 liters
   B. 27 liters
   C. 32 liters
   D. 40 liters
   E. 45 liters

237. The serum osmolarity is maintained at a concentration around 285 mOsm/L determined mainly by concentrations of sodium, chloride, and
   A. bicarbonate
   B. protein
   C. glucose
   D. magnesium
   E. potassium

238. Signs of severe dehydration include oliguria, hypotension, poor skin turgor, and a urine sodium of
A. > 20 mEq/L
B. > 30 mEq/L
C. < 40 mEq/L
D. < 10 mEq/L
E. < 30 mEq/L

239. Electrocardiographic abnormalities of hypokalemia include a prolonged QT interval, ST segment depression, and
A. peaked T waves
B. U waves
C. normal T wave duration
D. prolonged PR interval
E. V waves

240. One of the most common etiologies of loss of sodium in excess of body water resulting in hyponatremia is
A. diuretics
B. Addison disease
C. cirrhosis
D. renal failure
E. myxedema

241. One of the most common causes of water loss in excess of sodium loss resulting in hypernatremia is
A. uremia
B. methoxyflurane anesthesia
C. multiple myeloma
D. vomiting
E. dialysis

242. Pancreatitis, renal failure, pseudohypoparathyroidism, and hypomagnesemia all can cause
A. hypernatremia
B. hypercalcemia
C. metabolic alkalosis
D. hypokalemia
E. hypocalcemia

243. Loop diuretics, phosphate, calcitonin, steroids, and mithramycin are all medications that can be used in the treatment of
   A. hypocalcemia
   B. hypernatremia
   C. hyponatremia
   D. hypercalcemia
   E. hyperkalemia

244. In metabolic acidosis, one will see a decrease in pH and the following abnormalities
   A. $\uparrow$[H+], $\downarrow$Pco$_2$ and $\uparrow$Hco$_{3-}$
   B. $\downarrow$[H+], $\downarrow$Pco$_2$ and $\downarrow$Hco$_{3-}$
   C. $\uparrow$[H+], $\downarrow$Pco$_2$ and $\downarrow$Hco$_{3-}$
   D. $\uparrow$[H+], $\uparrow$Pco$_2$ and $\uparrow$Hco$_{3-}$
   E. $\downarrow$[H+], $\uparrow$Pco$_2$ and $\downarrow$Hco$_3$

245. Potassium chloride, fluids, and carbonic anhydrase inhibitors (acetazolamide) are all used to treat
   A. metabolic acidosis
   B. respiratory acidosis
   C. respiratory alkalosis
   D. hypernatremia
   E. metabolic alkalosis

Fluids, Electrolytes, and Acid–Base Balance

ANSWERS AND DISCUSSION

236. **(C)** The average 70-kg man contains 49 liters of water of which 32 liters is intracellular fluid and 5 liters is blood. **(Ref: *Essential Otolaryngology*, p. 359)**

237. **(A)** Protein and glucose contribute minimally to serum osmolarity except in cases of paraproteinemia and hyperglycemia. **(Ref: *Essential Otolaryngology*, pp. 360–361)**

238. **(D)** Other signs of dehydration include tachycardia and hemoconcentration. This is very important to be aware of, especially postoperatively. **(Ref: *Essential Otolaryngology*, pp. 359–360)**

239. **(B)** With hyperkalemia, there are peaked T waves, prolonged QRS, sinus arrest, and ventricular sine wave. With hypocalcemia, there is lengthened QT segment and normal T wave duration and with hypercalcemia there is a shortened QT interval. **(Ref: *Essential Otolaryngology*, pp. 364–365)**

240. **(A)** Other conditions that can result in hyponatremia include nephritis and osmotic diuresis. Extrarenal losses include vomiting, diarrhea, and third space losses. Addison disease, myxedema, and inappropriate antidiuretic syndrome can result in hyponatremia due to excess water. Congestive heart failure, nephrosis, cirrhosis, and renal failure can result in hyponatremia due to excess sodium and excess water. **(Ref: *Essential Otolaryngology*, pp. 362–363)**

241. (D) This is very important postoperatively. Other causes of water loss in excess of sodium loss include central or nephrogenic diabetes insipidus, diarrhea, severe burns, osmotic diuresis (calcium, glucose, IVP dye), and excessive insensible losses. **(Ref: *Essential Otolaryngology*, pp. 362–363)**

242. (E) Other causes of hypocalcemia may include hypomagnesemia, vitamin D deficiency, malabsorption, and hypoalbuminemia. **(Ref: *Essential Otolaryngology*, p. 600)**

243. (D) Conditions that can cause hypercalcemia are hyperparathyroidism, ectopic parathyroid hormone secretion, bony metastases, milk alkali syndrome, vitamin D toxicity, sarcoid, and tuberculosis. **(Ref: *Essential Otolaryngology*, pp. 601–602)**

244. (C) One of the most common causes of metabolic acidosis is diabetic ketoacidosis. Other causes of increased organic acid production include lactic acidosis, starvation ketosis, and alcoholic ketoacidosis. There are also numerous other causes of metabolic acidosis. **(Ref: *Essential Otolaryngology*, pp. 368–369)**

245. (E) The causes of metabolic alkalosis include diuretics, vomiting, diarrhea, antacid therapy, hyperaldosteronism, and gastrointestinal fistula. **(Ref: *Essential Otolaryngology*, pp. 370–371)**

19

Surgical Hemostasis

DIRECTIONS (Questions 246 through 265): Each of the numbered items or incomplete statements in this section is followed by answers or completions of the statement. Select the ONE lettered answer or completion that is BEST in each case.

---

246. The following factor is involved in the extrinsic system of coagulation
   A. VII
   B. XII
   C. IX
   D. V
   E. XIII

247. Platelet adhesion to collagen and subendothelial surfaces is in part dependent on normal synthesis of this factor by subendothelial cells and in megakaryocytes
   A. IX
   B. VIII
   C. XII
   D. V
   E. XIII

248. A 12-year-old boy is being worked up preoperatively for routine tonsillectomy. The screening tests for coagulation are all normal except the bleeding time is increased. One would suspect
    A. vitamin K deficiency
    B. liver disease
    C. factor VII deficiency
    D. platelet dysfunction
    E. factor IX deficiency

249. A 20-year-old female has an elevated PT and PTT and decreased factors IX and VII. She has
    A. hemophilia B
    B. vitamin K deficiency
    C. Von Willebrand disease
    D. thrombocytopenia
    E. factor IX deficiency

250. On a 15-year-old female, the platelet count is decreased and the bleeding time was increased. All other tests are normal. The most likely diagnosis is
    A. thrombocytopenia
    B. vitamin K deficiency
    C. DIC
    D. factor XII deficiency
    E. hemophilia B

251. The following medication has been used in certain types of Von Willebrand disease
    A. vitamin K
    B. vitamin D
    C. DDAVP
    D. Inderol
    E. BBVD

252. An inherited disease of the lysosomal membrane of granulocytes is
    A. agranulocytosis
    B. porphyrias
    C. polycythemia
    D. megaloblastic anemia
    E. Chédiak–Higashi disease

253. A 15-year-old female has normal PT and PTT but a bone marrow shows an increased number of megakaryocytes. The most likely diagnosis is
A. agranulocytosis
B. polycythemia
C. megaloblastic anemia
D. idiopathic thrombocytopenia
E. factor IX deficiency

254. A 50-year-old male who is an alcoholic with chronic liver disease presents with photosensitive vesicles of the skin and oral mucous membranes. He most likely has
A. porphyria cutanea tarda
B. uremia
C. vitamin K deficiency
D. DIC
E. platelet dysfunction

255. A 60-year-old male presents with dysphagia, atrophic glossitis, koilonychia, and anemia. He most likely has
A. agranulocytosis
B. Plummer–Vinson syndrome
C. porphyria
D. thrombocytopenia
E. vitamin K deficiency

256. The PTT test is most sensitive to abnormalities and deficiency of factors involved prior to activation of factor
A. XII
B. XI
C. IX
D. VIII
E. X

257. Low levels of fibrinogen (factor I) may be seen in DIC, fibrinolysis, and
A. vitamin K deficiency
B. severe liver disease
C. Von Willebrand disease
D. hemophilia A
E. uremia

258. A prolonged thrombin time in the face of a normal reptilase time suggests
  A. vitamin K deficiency
  B. liver disease
  C. heparin effect
  D. DIC
  E. hemophilia A

259. A 40-year-old male has severe thrombocytopenia. One would consider prophylactically treating this man with platelets if his platelet count fell to less than
  A. 20,000 mm^3
  B. 40,000 mm^3
  C. 60,000 mm^3
  D. 80,000 mm^3
  E. 100,000 mm^3

260. Ristocetin cofactor measures the functional activity in
  A. factor XII deficiency
  B. vitamin K deficiency
  C. hemophilia B
  D. Von Willebrand disease
  E. factor XI deficiency

261. The following condition is a chronic anemia that can present as an oral cavity mass caused by extramedullary hematopoiesis
  A. Chédiak–Higashi disease
  B. thalassemia
  C. Plummer–Vinson disease
  D. agranulocytosis
  E. Von Willebrand disease

262. DDAVP can be fatal if used in the following situation
  A. type I Von Willebrand disease
  B. type II A Von Willebrand
  C. type II B Von Willebrand
  D. can be used on all Von Willebrand
  E. cannot be used on Von Willebrand

263. The presence of a low factor VIII level and a normal factor VIII-related antigen suggests classic
   A. hemophilia A
   B. hemophilia B
   C. vitamin K deficiency
   D. factor XII deficiency
   E. factor V deficiency

264. A 40-year-old male presents to your office after ileum resection surgery with painful atrophy of the entire oral mucous membrane and tongue as well as recurrent aphthous ulcers. An appropriate test to order would be a
   A. vitamin B_{12} level
   B. folate level
   C. vitamin K level
   D. factor IX level
   E. factor VIII level

265. The following medication is a fibrinolytic inhibitor and can be used for hemophilia
   A. DDAVP
   B. EACA
   C. Inderol
   D. vitamin K
   E. AquaMephyton

Surgical Hemostasis

ANSWERS AND DISCUSSION

246. (A) The extrinsic system of coagulation is initiated by tissue damage, which activates tissue thromboplastin and this activates factor VII. (**Ref:** *Essential Otolaryngology*, **p. 342**)

247. (B) Von Willebrand disease is a dominantly inherited disease of the intrinsic pathway. (**Ref:** *Otolaryngology—Head and Neck Surgery*, **p. 1223**)

248. (D) This would be typical of platelet dysfunction. (**Ref:** *Essential Otolaryngology*, **p. 343**)

249. (B) This is typical of vitamin K deficiency. (**Ref:** *Essential Otolaryngology*, **p. 343**)

250. (A) This is consistent with thrombocytopenia. (**Ref:** *Essential Otolaryngology*, **p. 343**)

251. (C) Arginine vasopression (DDAVP) has been used to treat certain types of Von Willebrand disease to obviate the need for blood component therapy. (**Ref:** *Otolaryngology—Head and Neck Surgery*, **p. 1223**)

252. (E) Chédiak–Higashi disease is an inherited disease of the lysosomal membrane of granuloctyes, characterized by large blue lysosomal particles in white cells demonstrated with Wright stain. **(Ref: *Otolaryngology—Head and Neck Surgery,* p. 1223)**

253. (D) Idiopathic thrombocytopenia is an immunologic disorder in which platelets are first sensitized and then destroyed by the spleen or liver. Most cases remit spontaneously and require no specific treatment. **(Ref: *Pediatric Otolaryngology,* p. 938)**

254. (A) This is typical of porphyria cutanea tarda and results in defects in the metabolic assembly of the hemoglobin molecule. **(Ref: *Otolaryngology—Head and Neck Surgery,* p. 1223)**

255. (B) Plummer–Vinson syndrome is a symptom complex caused by iron deficiency and also there are associated esophageal webs. **(Ref: *Otolaryngology—Head and Neck Surgery,* p. 1222)**

256. (E) PTT evaluates all the coagulation factors in the intrinsic coagulation system and final common pathway. **(Ref: *Essential Otolaryngology,* p. 344)**

257. (B) Severe liver disease can cause a decrease in fibrinogen. **(Ref: *Essential Otolaryngology,* p. 344)**

258. (C) This is an excellent way to test for heparin effect. **(Ref: *Essential Otolaryngology,* p. 345)**

259. (A) As well, all patients with hemorrhage and thrombocytopenia are given platelet transfusions. A unit of random donor platelets concentrate can be expected to raise the platelet count by $10,000/mm^3/m^2$ of body surface area. **(Ref: *Essential Otolaryngology,* p. 346)**

260. (D) Factor VIII-related antigen measures the level of Von Willebrand factor in plasma and ristocetin cofactor measures the functional activity of Von Willebrand factor. **(Ref: *Essential Otolaryngology,* p. 348)**

261. (B) Thalassemia can present as an oral cavity mass or as a prominent maxilla with severe malocclusion. (**Ref:** *Otolaryngology—Head and Neck Surgery,* **p. 1223**)

262. (C) If one uses DDAVP, one has to make a precise diagnosis of the type of variant as type II B can be followed by severe thrombocytopenia after use of DDAVP. (**Ref:** *Essential Otolaryngology,* **p. 349**)

263. (A) Low levels of factor VIII antigen and ristocetin cofactor suggest Von Willebrand disease. (**Ref:** *Essential Otolaryngology,* **p. 349**)

264. (A) Patients with megaloblastic anemia from B_{12} deficiency present sometimes with this "magenta tongue." (**Ref:** *Otolaryngology—Head and Neck Surgery,* **p. 1223**)

265. (B) The fibrinolytic inhibitor EACA can be administered in conjunction with factor replacement, primarily when patients are undergoing oral surgery and dental extractions. (**Ref:** *Essential Otolaryngology,* **p. 351**)

20

Cancer Chemotherapy

DIRECTIONS (Questions 266 through 275): Each of the numbered items or incomplete statements in this section is followed by answers or completions of the statement. Select the ONE lettered answer or completion that is BEST in each case.

266. Cisplatin is used for lung and head and neck cancers. It is a chemotherapeutic agent that is in the class of
    A. alkylating agents
    B. nitrosoureas
    C. antimetabolites
    D. mitotic inhibitors
    E. antihormonal agents

267. This chemotherapeutic agent used to treat testicular and lung cancer can be very ototoxic. It is
    A. busulfan
    B. ifusfamide
    C. cyclophosphamide
    D. carboplatin
    E. melphalan

268. This group of chemotherapeutic agents are lipid soluble and behave like alkylating agents. They are used in treatment of primary brain tumors. They are
   A. hormones
   B. nitrosoureas
   C. antimetabolites
   D. mitotic inhibitors
   E. antihormones

269. Methotrexate is a
   A. pyrimidine analog
   B. purine analog
   C. folic acid antagonist
   D. hormone
   E. alkylating agent

270. A 50-year-old female has breast cancer and is placed in this regime of chemotherapy but develops ataxia as a side effect. The agent is
   A. hydroxyurea
   B. semustine
   C. triazinate
   D. 5-fluorouracil
   E. floxuridine

271. This 5-year-old male is being treated for leukemia. He develops alopecia. This is a most common complication of
   A. methotrexate
   B. 5-fluorouracil
   C. doxorubicin
   D. levamisole
   E. procarbazine

272. A 20-year-old male has Hodgkin disease. He had positive lymph nodes in regions on both sides of the diaphragm. He is classified as a
   A. stage I
   B. stage II

C. stage III
D. stage IV
E. stage IV$_E$

273. A 30-year-old female patient with Hodgkin disease has localized involvement of contiguous extralymphatic sites and one other lymph node region in the same side of the diaphragm. She is classified as
A. stage I
B. stage II
C. stage II$_E$
D. stage III
E. stage III$_E$

274. The standard therapy for chemotherapy for Hodgkin disease is
A. MOPP
B. CBM
C. dactinomycin
D. fludarabine
E. vinblastine

275. According to this classification, a lymphoblastic lymphoma would fall in the high grade category. This classification is that of
A. Mustarde
B. Rappaport
C. DeVita
D. Schein
E. Noble

Cancer Chemotherapy

ANSWERS AND DISCUSSION

266. (A) Cisplatin is an alkylating agent that is also used in the treatment of testicular and ovarian cancers. **(Ref: *Essential Otolaryngology*, pp. 397–398)**

267. (D) Carboplatin can be toxic to the ear as well as having bone marrow suppression. **(Ref: *Essential Otolaryngology*, p. 398)**

268. (B) Nitrosoureas gain access to the central nervous system but are also used in treatment of lymphomas and myeloma. **(Ref: *Essential Otolaryngology*, p. 400)**

269. (C) Methotrexate to date has been the single most used drug in the treatment of carcinomas of the head and neck. It is an antimetabolite. **(Ref: *Essential Otolaryngology*, p. 396)**

270. (D) Ataxia can be a common CNS complication of 5-fluorouracil. **(Ref: *Essential Otolaryngology*, p. 396)**

271. (C) Doxorubicin and daunorubicin are known to cause alopecia. **(Ref: *Essential Otolaryngology*, p. 401)**

272. (C) According to the Ann Arbor Staging System, he would be classified as a stage III. **(Ref: *Essential Otolaryngology*, p. 883)**

273. **(C)** According to the Ann Arbor Staging System, she would be classified as a stage II_E. **(Ref: *Essential Otolaryngology*, p. 883)**

274. **(A)** The standard treatment for Hodgkin disease is MOPP, which consists of mechlorethamine, vincristine, procarbazine, and prednisone. **(Ref: *Essential Otolaryngology*, p. 883)**

275. **(B)** Rappaport classified non-Hodgkin lymphoma into low grade, intermediate grade, and high grade. Since then, they have been reclassified by an Expert International Panel into a working formulation of non-Hodgkin lymphoma for clinical use. **(Ref: *Essential Otolaryngology*, p. 883)**

21

Nasal Endoscopy and Its Surgical Applications

DIRECTIONS (Questions 276 through 290): Each of the numbered items or incomplete statements in this section is followed by answers or completions of the statement. Select the ONE lettered answer or completion that is BEST in each case.

---

276. The incidence of accessary ostia from the maxillary sinus is approximately
    A. 10 to 20%
    B. 20 to 30%
    C. 30 to 40%
    D. 40 to 50%
    E. 50 to 60%

277. The Onodi cell is
    A. a rare cell found in the middle turbinate
    B. the most lateral cell of the anterior ethmoid cells
    C. the most posterior of the posterior ethmoid cells
    D. is the cell that invaginates anteriorly into the anterior ethmoid cells
    E. is the cell that indents the inferior wall of the frontal sinus

278. A clinical bony dehiscence of the cavernous portion of the carotid canal is present in the following percentage of patients
   A. 2%
   B. 5%
   C. 10%
   D. 22%
   E. 35%

279. As a landmark, one uses the anterior ethmoid artery. It is important to know that this can be absent unilaterally in the following percentage of patients
   A. 2%
   B. 5%
   C. 14%
   D. 20%
   E. 25%

280. The range of bacteria involved in acute sinusitis include *Streptococcus pneumoniae, Staphylococcus aureus, Hemophilus influenzae,* and
   A. bacteroids
   B. *Streptococcus pyogenes*
   C. *Neisseria* sp
   D. *Escherichia coli*
   E. corynebacteria

281. The most common fungal sinus infection in an otherwise healthy patient is
   A. *Candida albicans*
   B. veillonella
   C. peptostreptococci
   D. *Aspergillus niger*
   E. corynebacteria

282. Woodworkers have an increased incidence of this type of tumor in the maxillary sinus
   A. adenocarcinoma
   B. squamous cell carcinoma
   C. adenoid cystic carcinoma
   D. malignant mixed carcinoma
   E. acinic cell carcinoma

283. An anatomic variation of the ethmoidal infundibulum can be related to the following cells
   A. lamellar cell
   B. Haller cell
   C. Onodi cell
   D. frontal cell
   E. agger nasi cell

284. The most common sinus involved in inflammatory sinus disease is the
   A. sphenoid sinus
   B. frontal sinus
   C. ethmoid sinus
   D. maxillary sinus
   E. sphenoid and frontal sinuses

285. A 30-year-old immunosuppressed female had a CT scan that showed metallic densities within the maxillary sinus. Another test that may be helpful would be a
   A. T_2-weighted MRI
   B. bone scan
   C. CBC with diff.
   D. echogram
   E. repeat CT scan with contrast

286. Squamous cell carcinoma is the most common true neoplasm of the paranasal sinus. The incidence is approximately
   A. 1:20,000
   B. 1:50,000
   C. 1:150,000
   D. 1:200,000
   E. 1:400,000

287. The incidence of CSF rhinorrhea in patients who suffer serious head trauma is
   A. < 1%
   B. 2 to 3%
   C. 5%
   D. 10%
   E. 20%

288. The most common postoperative complication of endoscopic sinus surgery is
  A. orbital emphysema
  B. CSF leak
  C. orbital hematoma
  D. synechia
  E. epiphora

289. The following percentage of patients with CSF rhinorrhea develop meningitis as their initial symptom
  A. 2%
  B. 10%
  C. 20%
  D. 30%
  E. 40%

290. The following laser can be helpful with massive polyposis to reduce blood loss
  A. tunable dye laser
  B. pulsed dye laser
  C. KTP/532 laser
  D. CO_2 laser
  E. copper vapor laser

Nasal Endoscopy and Its Surgical Applications

ANSWERS AND DISCUSSION

276. (B) Approximately 20 to 30% of maxillary sinuses have an accessory ostia and it is important to recognize this as one should open the natural ostia in order to get proper drainage. **(Ref: *Essential Otolaryngology*, p. 374)**

277. (C) This Onodi cell is the most posterior cell of the posterior ethmoid sinuses and is often lateral to and well behind the anterior face of the sphenoid sinus. **(Ref: *Essential Otolaryngology*, p. 375)**

278. (D) A clinical bony dehiscence is present in approximately 22% of patients. This is extremely important clinically. **(Ref: *Essential Otolaryngology*, p. 375)**

279. (C) The anterior ethmoid artery is absent unilaterally in approximately 14% of patients and is bilaterally absent in 2% of patients. **(Ref: *Essential Otolaryngology*, p. 375)**

280. (B) The range of organisms is different for acute and chronic sinusitis. **(Ref: *Otolaryngology—Head and Neck Surgery*, pp. 956–957)**

281. (D) Aspergillosis is the most common fungus found in an otherwise healthy patient. **(Ref: *Otolaryngology—Head and Neck Surgery*, p. 957)**

282. (A) Woodworkers have an increased incidence of adenocarcinoma and nickel workers have an increased incidence of squamous cell carcinoma of the maxillary sinus. **(Ref: *Essential Otolaryngology*, p. 376)**

283. (B) The presence of a Haller cell can cause a variation of the ethmoidal infundibulum. **(Ref: *Essential Otolaryngology*, p. 376)**

284. (C) Of patients with inflammatory sinus disease, 93% had sinus disease in the ethmoid while 79% had inflammatory disease in the maxillary sinus. **(Ref: *Essential Otolaryngology*, p. 378)**

285. (A) In this situation, an MRI scan is helpful as the T_2-weighted image will reveal a reduced signal intensity in a patient with fungal sinus disease. **(Ref: *Essential Otolaryngology*, p. 379)**

286. (D) Malignancy in the paranasal sinus is not common and it usually mimics benign disease initially. **(Ref: *Otolaryngology—Head and Neck Surgery*, p. 941)**

287. (B) Only 2 to 3% of patients who suffer serious head trauma have CSF rhinorrhea but accidental trauma is the cause of 80% of the patients with CSF rhinorrhea. **(Ref: *Otolaryngology—Head and Neck Surgery*, p. 965)**

288. (D) By far, synechia is the most common complication of endoscopic sinus surgery. The prevention of this is aided by careful postoperative follow-up and nasal cleaning. **(Ref: *Essential Otolaryngology*, p. 386)**

289. (C) Approximately 20% of patients with CSF rhinorrhea develop meningitis as their initial manifestation. **(Ref: *Otolaryngology—Head and Neck Surgery*, p. 967)**

290. (C) The KTP/532 laser can help but generally complete laser obliteration of nasal polyposis is impractical and too time consuming. **(Ref: *Essential Otolaryngology*, p. 385)**

22

Antimicrobial Therapy in Head and Neck Surgery

DIRECTIONS (Questions 291 through 305): Each of the numbered items or incomplete statements in this section is followed by answers or completions of the statement. Select the ONE lettered answer or completion that is BEST in each case.

291. In the general population, the incidence of anaphylaxis as a result of the use of penicillin-based antibiotics is
   A. 1:2000
   B. 1:5000
   C. 1:10,000
   D. 1:50,000
   E. 1:100,000

292. The incidence of a rash as a result of penicillin use is as high as
   A. 0.5%
   B. 1%
   C. 2%
   D. 5%
   E. 10%

293. Ampicillin is active against all of the following organisms except
   A. *H. influenzae*
   B. *E. coli*
   C. *Streptococcus pyogenes*
   D. *Streptococcus pneumoniae*
   E. *Staphylococcus aureus*

294. One of the major side effects of long-term isoniazid treatment is
   A. aplastic anemia
   B. peripheral neuropathy
   C. leukopenia
   D. seizures
   E. erythema multiforme

295. Cephalexin has very poor coverage against
   A. *Staphylococcus aureus*
   B. *Streptococcus*
   C. *H. influenzae*
   D. *E. coli*
   E. *Proteus*

296. Cefuroxime has good coverage against
   A. *H. influenzae*
   B. *Streptococcus*
   C. *Pneumococcus*
   D. *Bacteroides*
   E. *Neisseria gonorrhoeae*

297. The following antibiotic can significantly elevate theophylline levels in the bloodstream
   A. clindamycin
   B. cefixime
   C. erythromycin
   D. ticarcillin
   E. tetracycline

298. The following antibiotic suspension has been helpful against aphthous stomatitis
- **A.** vancomycin
- **B.** clindamycin
- **C.** erythromycin
- **D.** tetracycline
- **E.** chloramphenicol

299. The incidence of fatal bone marrow suspension with the use of chloramphenicol is approximately
- **A.** 1:1000
- **B.** 1:5000
- **C.** 1:10,000
- **D.** 1:24,000
- **E.** 1:85,000

300. Ciprofloxacin is very active against the following organisms except
- **A.** *Pseudomonas aeruginosa*
- **B.** *Staphylococcus aureus*
- **C.** *H. influenzae*
- **D.** *Bacteroides fragiles*
- **E.** *Streptococcus pyogenes*

301. The following is very effective against *Legionella pneumophilia*
- **A.** chloramphenicol
- **B.** clindamycin
- **C.** vancomycin
- **D.** erythromycin
- **E.** tetracycline

302. The following medication exerts its antibacterial activity via the inhibition of bacterial topoisomerase II
- **A.** ciprofloxacin
- **B.** imipenem
- **C.** vancomycin
- **D.** chloramphenicol
- **E.** clindamycin

303. With long-term amphotericin administration, one should monitor
    A. renal function
    B. hepatic function
    C. bone marrow
    D. PT, PTT
    E. cardiac status

304. The following medication is effective against intestinal parasites
    A. vancomycin
    B. chloramphenicol
    C. mebendazole
    D. clindamycin
    E. fluconazole

305. The following medication can be ototoxic in high doses
    A. rifampin
    B. amphotericin B
    C. ketoconazole
    D. ciprofloxacin
    E. vancomycin

Antimicrobial Therapy in Head and Neck Surgery

ANSWERS AND DISCUSSION

291. (C) In the general population, the incidence of anaphylaxis with penicillin use is 1:10,000. (**Ref:** *Essential Otolaryngology,* **p. 390**)

292. (D) The incidence of a rash from penicillin use can be as high as 5%; however, the next exposure to penicillin may result in an anaphylactic reaction in some patients. (**Ref:** *Essential Otolaryngology,* **p. 389**)

293. (E) One of the major drawbacks of ampicillin and amoxil is its resistance to *Staphylococcus aureus,* a 20% resistance to *H. influenzae,* and a 75% resistance to *Branhamella catarrhalis.* (**Ref:** *Essential Otolaryngology,* **p. 390**)

294. (B) Isoniazid, metronidazole, and nitrofurantoin can all be associated with peripheral neuropathy. (**Ref:** *Otolaryngology—Head and Neck Surgery,* **p. 106**)

295. (C) Cephalexin is active against *Staphylococcus aureus, Streptococcus, Pneumococcus, E. coli, Proteus,* and *Klebsiella.* It has poor coverage against *Hemophilus, Pseudomonas,* and *Bacteroides.* (**Ref:** *Essential Otolaryngology,* **p. 391**)

296. (D) One of the drawbacks of second generation cephalosporins is the poor coverage against *Pseudomonas* and *Bacteroides*. **(Ref: *Essential Otolaryngology*, p. 391)**

297. (C) Erythromycin can significantly elevate theophylline levels. **(Ref: *Essential Otolaryngology*, p. 393)**

298. (D) Tetracycline suspension may help in aphthous stomatitis. **(Ref: *Essential Otolaryngology*, p. 393)**

299. (D) With chloramphenicol use, the incidence of aplastic anemia is an idiosyncratic, nondose-related mechanism that has an even higher incidence with oral administration. **(Ref: *Otolaryngology—Head and Neck Surgery*, p. 111)**

300. (D) Ciprofloxacin has poor activity against anaerobes. **(Ref: *Essential Otolaryngology*, p. 394)**

301. (D) Intravenous therapy with erythromycin has been reserved primarily for patients who are severely infected with the *Legionella* species. **(Ref: *Otolaryngology—Head and Neck Surgery*, p. 111)**

302. (A) Ciprofloxacin is in the quinoline group of medications and has no activity against anaerobes. **(Ref: *Otolaryngology—Head and Neck Surgery*, p. 112)**

303. (A) Patients treated with amphotericin B on a long-term basis will often experience mild renal impairment, which may lead to permanent renal damage. **(Ref: *Otolaryngology—Head and Neck Surgery*, p. 113)**

304. (C) Mebendazole is an antiparasitic agent that will provide broad-spectrum antiparasitic therapy. **(Ref: *Otolaryngology—Head and Neck Surgery*, p. 113)**

305. (E) Vancomycin can be toxic and nephrotoxic if it is given in high doses. **(Ref: *Essential Otolaryngology*, p. 395)**

23

Nutritional Assessment and Support

DIRECTIONS (Questions 306 through 315): Each of the numbered items or incomplete statements in this section is followed by answers or completions of the statement. Select the ONE lettered answer or completion that is BEST in each case.

306. One of the earliest indications that there are changes in protein malnutrition is the serum level of
    A. transferrin
    B. Hgb
    C. Cr
    D. SGPT
    E. carotene

307. Serum albumin level decreases are indicative of malnutrition. One has severe malnutrition if the serum albumin level is less than
    A. 5.0
    B. 4.0
    C. 3.5
    D. 3.0
    E. 2.0

308. Serum total lymphocyte/mm³ levels are correlated with nutrition. One has severe malnutrition if the level falls below
   A. 5000
   B. 3000
   C. 2000
   D. 1200
   E. 800

309. Clinical indicators of malnutrition are a change in weight of
   A. 5%
   B. 10%
   C. 15%
   D. 20%
   E. 25%

310. The most common complication of tube feeding is
   A. aspiration
   B. bloating
   C. renal compromise
   D. diarrhea
   E. esophageal irritation

311. With peripheral parenteral nutrition, the percentage of amino acids should be approximately
   A. 1%
   B. 2%
   C. 3.5%
   D. 10%
   E. 20%

312. The catabolic patient requires the following calories per gram of nitrogen for tissue synthesis in the composition of the central parenteral solution
   A. 50 to 100
   B. 100 to 150
   C. 150 to 200
   D. 200 to 250
   E. 250 to 300

313. Fats are important in central parenteral solutions. They are given as a fatty acid solution in the following concentration
  A. 5 to 10%
  B. 10 to 20%
  C. 20 to 30%
  D. 30 to 40%
  E. 50%

314. Ensure contains the following amount of calories per mL
  A. 0.5
  B. 0.75
  C. 1.06
  D. 2.32
  E. 4.8

315. Serum transferrin levels are linked to malnutrition. One has severe malnutrition if the serum transferrin level is less than
  A. 300 mg/dL
  B. 200 mg/dL
  C. 175 mg/dL
  D. 150 mg/dL
  E. 100 mg/dL

Nutritional Assessment and Support

ANSWERS AND DISCUSSION

306. (A) Transferrin serum level measurement reflects early evidence of protein malnutrition as well as the earliest indication of its reversal. (**Ref:** *Essential Otolaryngology,* **p. 400**)

307. (E) Serum albumin levels of less than 2.0 are indicative of severe malnutrition. (**Ref:** *Otolaryngology—Head and Neck Surgery,* **p. 1673**)

308. (E) Serum total lymphocyte levels of less than 800 reflect severe malnutrition. (**Ref:** *Otolaryngology—Head and Neck Surgery,* **p. 1673**)

309. (C) Weight change of 15%, weight that is less than 80% of the patient's usual predisease weight, and weight of less than 85% of the ideal body weight are all indicators of malnutrition. (**Ref:** *Otolaryngology—Head and Neck Surgery,* **p. 1674**)

310. (D) Diarrhea is the most common complication of tube feedings and can be related to a hypoalbuminemia or an overly rapid rate of administration. (**Ref:** *Otolaryngology—Head and Neck Surgery,* **p. 1676**)

311. **(C)** The preferred method of reducing the catabolic state is to give 5 to 10% dextrose and 3.5% amino acids for a total of approximately 2000 cc per day with intralipid to increase the total caloric intake. (**Ref:** *Essential Otolaryngology*, **p. 401**)

312. **(B)** The catabolic patient requires 100 to 150 calories per gram of nitrogen for tissue synthesis. (**Ref:** *Essential Otolaryngology*, **p. 402**)

313. **(B)** Fats are given in tandem as a 10 to 20% fatty acid solution. (**Ref:** *Essential Otolaryngology*, **p. 401**)

314. **(C)** Ensure contains 1.06 calories per mL and 37.2 grams of protein per liter. (**Ref:** *Otolaryngology—Head and Neck Surgery*, **p. 1674**)

315. **(E)** The serum transferrin level of less than 175 mg/dL indicates mild malnutrition. Levels less than 100 mg/dL indicate severe malnutrition. (**Ref:** *Otolaryngology—Head and Neck Surgery*, **p. 1673**)

24

Neck Spaces and Facial Planes

DIRECTIONS (Questions 316 through 320): Each of the numbered items or incomplete statements in this section is followed by answers or completions of the statement. Select the ONE lettered answer or completion that is BEST in each case.

316. In draining an abscess in the occipital triangle, one has to be careful not to traumatize the following cranial nerve
    A. X
    B. IX
    C. XII
    D. VII
    E. XI

317. The strap muscles of the neck are enveloped in the
    A. deep layer of the deep cervical fascia
    B. middle layer of the deep cervical fascia
    C. superficial layer of the deep cervical fascia
    D. superficial cervical fascia
    E. carotid sheath

318. The lateral pharyngeal space is divided into two compartments by the
  - **A.** XIth cranial nerve
  - **B.** carotid artery
  - **C.** deep layer of the deep cervical fascia
  - **D.** styloid process
  - **E.** jugular artery

319. The most common source of infection of the lateral pharyngeal space is from the
  - **A.** soft palate
  - **B.** mastoid
  - **C.** tonsil
  - **D.** neck
  - **E.** floor of mouth

320. The hallmark of actinomycosis is a chronic granuloma with
  - **A.** ferritin deposits
  - **B.** large blast cells
  - **C.** Reid–Sternberg cells
  - **D.** eosinophil proliferation
  - **E.** sulfur granules

Neck Spaces and Facial Planes

ANSWERS AND DISCUSSION

316. **(E)** The occipital triangle is defined anteriorly by the sternoclei-domastoid muscle, posteriorly by the trapezius muscle, and inferiorly by the omohyoid muscle. The XIth cranial nerve lies very superficially in this space. (**Ref:** *Essential Otolaryngology,* **p. 407**)

317. **(B)** The middle layer of the deep cervical fascia forms the pretracheal fascia, which overlies the trachea and buccopharyngeal fascia, which lies in the pharyngeal wall. Buccopharyngeal fascia forms a midline raphe in the posterior midline, which adheres to the prevertebral fascia, and a pterygomandibular raphe in the lateral pharynx. (**Ref:** *Essential Otolaryngology,* **p. 408**)

318. **(D)** This space is a very common source of infection extending from a peritonsillar abscess. Direct extension can also occur from the parotid, submandibular, retropharyngeal, masticator, and carotid sheath spaces. (**Ref:** *Essential Otolaryngology,* **p. 410**)

319. **(C)** Every peritonsillar space abscess is a potential pharyngomaxillary abscess. Other sources of infection include the pharynx, the teeth, the petrous portion of the temporal bone, the parotid gland (deep lobe), and the lymph nodes that drain the nose and the pharynx. (**Ref:** *Essential Otolaryngology,* **p. 410**)

320. (E) *Actinomyces* is a bacterium that is a gram-positive bacillus which often branches, giving it a fungal appearance. Diagnosis is best made by biopsy since the bacillus is fastidious and hard to grow. Penicillin is the drug of choice and should be given for a period of 6 to 12 months. (**Ref:** *Essential Otolaryngology,* **p. 421**)

25

The Oral Cavity, Oropharynx, and Hypopharynx

DIRECTIONS (Questions 321 through 340): Each of the numbered items or incomplete statements in this section is followed by answers or completions of the statement. Select the ONE lettered answer or completion that is BEST in each case.

321. The general visceral afferents of touch and gag sensation project to nucleus solitarius of the
    A. cerebellum
    B. cortex
    C. medulla
    D. pons
    E. thalamus

322. The lingual artery comes off the external carotid as the branch number
    A. 1
    B. 2
    C. 3
    D. 4
    E. 5

323. No taste buds are present in the following papillae
  A. fungiform
  B. foliate
  C. filiform
  D. filiform and foliate
  E. foliate and fungiform

324. The first molar erupts at approximately
  A. 10 months
  B. 12 months
  C. 15 months
  D. 20 months
  E. 22 months

325. The tensor veli palatini is innervated by
  A. V_3
  B. IX
  C. X
  D. VII
  E. V_2

326. The average amount of saliva produced in mL/day is
  A. 500
  B. 1000
  C. 1500
  D. 2000
  E. 2500

327. The condition in which the tooth root, as a result of trauma, fails to develop normally, resulting in an angular malformation of the root is called
  A. anodontia
  B. dilaceration
  C. enamel hypoplasia
  D. supernumerary teeth
  E. radicular tooth development

328. The organism cultured from acute necrotizing ulcerative gingivitis is
  A. *Borrelia vincentii*
  B. *Candida albicans*

C. *Peptococcus* sp
D. *Moraxella catarrhalis*
E. *Streptococcus viridans*

329. The syndrome of recurrent aphthous ulcers is called
    A. Smith disease
    B. Newman disease
    C. Koplik disease
    D. Sutton disease
    E. Peutz–Jegher syndrome

330. An 18-year-old male presents to your office with a slow-growing mandibular swelling. X-ray reveals a concentric (onion skin) layered appearance. The diagnosis is most likely
    A. ameloblastic sarcoma
    B. adenoameloblastoma
    C. cementoma
    D. odontoma
    E. Ewing sarcoma

331. A 12-year-old male has a dirty gray membrane on his tonsils, tonsillar pillars, and uvula. Attempts to remove it cause bleeding. There is also marked cervical adenopathy. Fluorescent antibody studies were done and shown to be positive. He has
    A. Vincent angina
    B. infectious mononucleosis
    C. scarlet fever
    D. diphtheria
    E. *Candida albicans* infection

332. The following percentage of sore throats is caused by group A beta-hemolytic streptococci
    A. 0 to 5%
    B. 5 to 10%
    C. 15 to 20%
    D. 20 to 30%
    E. 40 to 50%

333. The incidence of rheumatic fever with untreated acute streptococcal tonsillitis is
   A. 1%
   B. 3%
   C. 8%
   D. 10%
   E. 15%

334. A young child has had recurrent tonsillitis and a date is set for surgery. He is due to have a routine polio booster. One should
   A. delay surgery for 6 weeks after a polio vaccination
   B. not delay surgery
   C. delay surgery for 2 weeks after polio vaccination
   D. delay surgery for 12 weeks after polio vaccination
   E. delay polio booster until after tonsillectomy

335. The death rate from tonsillectomy is approximately
   A. 1:5000
   B. 1:7000
   C. 1:17,000
   D. 1:50,000
   E. 1:100,000

336. The incidence of primary hemorrhage after tonsillectomy is
   A. < 0.5%
   B. 0.5 to 2.2%
   C. 3 to 5%
   D. 5 to 7%
   E. 7 to 10%

337. The incidence of velopharyngeal insufficiency after T&A is between
   A. 1:100 and 1:500
   B. 1:750 and 1:1500
   C. 1:1500 and 1:2500
   D. 1:2500 and 1:5000
   E. > 1:5000

338. The incidence of nasopharyngeal cicatricial stenosis is
    A. 1:10,000
    B. 1:33,000
    C. 1:54,000
    D. 1:100,000
    E. 1:200,000

339. A 15-year-old male presents to your office with a severe sore throat and dysphagia. X-ray of the neck shows a widening of the soft tissue shadow over C2. This is pathologic if the width is more than
    A. 2 mm
    B. 4 mm
    C. 5 mm
    D. 6 mm
    E. 7 mm

340. In deep neck infections, sometimes there is no specific source of infection. The frequency of this is
    A. 10%
    B. 20%
    C. 30%
    D. 40%
    E. 50%

The Oral Cavity, Oropharynx, and Hypopharynx

ANSWERS AND DISCUSSION

321. (D) The afferents for touch and gag project to the nucleus solitarius of the pons. **(Ref:** *Essential Otolaryngology,* **p. 463)**

322. (B) The lingual artery is the second branch of the external carotid. **(Ref:** *Essential Otolaryngology,* **p. 463)**

323. (C) The filiform papillae contain no taste buds. These are present in the fungi form and foliate papillae. **(Ref:** *Essential Otolaryngology,* **p. 463)**

324. (C) The first molar erupts at approximately 15 months. This can contribute to otalgia at this time. **(Ref:** *Essential Otolaryngology,* **p. 463)**

325. (A) The mandibular nerve V_3 innervates the tensor palatini. The remainder of the palatal muscles are innervated by the pharyngeal plexus, IX and X. **(Ref:** *Essential Otolaryngology,* **p. 464)**

326. (C) Approximately 1500 mL/day of saliva is produced, with a pH between 6.2 and 7.4. **(Ref:** *Essential Otolaryngology,* **p. 465)**

327. (B) Dilaceration is associated with rickets and cretinism. **(Ref: Essential Otolaryngology, p. 465)**

328. (A) *Borrelia vincentii* is the organism cultured from Vincent angina. **(Ref: Essential Otolaryngology, p. 466)**

329. (D) The history of Sutton disease is multiple, large deep ulcers that cause extensive scarring in the oral cavity. **(Ref: Essential Otolaryngology, p. 466)**

330. (E) In 50% of patients, there is an onioned skin pattern on x-ray. The 5-year survival is less than 15%. **(Ref: Essential Otolaryngology, p. 469)**

331. (D) Identification of diphtheria is by fluorescent antibody studies. Also, the presence of Klebs–Loeffler bacillus in the membrane is diagnosed by Gram stain and culture. **(Ref: Otolaryngology—Head and Neck Surgery, p. 1181)**

332. (C) Approximately 15 to 20% of sore throats are caused by group A beta-hemolytic streptococci. **(Ref: Otolaryngology—Head and Neck Surgery, p. 1182)**

333. (B) Approximately 3% of untreated B-hemolytic *Streptococcus* infections of the tonsils can result in rheumatic fever. Acute glomerulonephritis can occur in 10 to 15% of patients after infection with certain serotypes. **(Ref: Otolaryngology—Head and Neck Surgery, p. 1185)**

334. (A) A delay of 6 weeks after vaccination is advisable because, in previous epidemics, poliomyelitis increased after tonsillectomy. **(Ref: Otolaryngology—Head and Neck Surgery, p. 1191)**

335. (C) Surprisingly, the death rate from tonsillectomy has been reported at approximately 1:17,000. **(Ref: Otolaryngology—Head and Neck Surgery, p. 1193)**

336. (B) The incidence of secondary hemorrhage can be as high as 3%. **(Ref: Otolaryngology—Head and Neck Surgery, p. 1193)**

337. **(B)** One should be very cautious if there is a submucous cleft palate or even a bifid uvula. **(Ref:** *Otolaryngology—Head and Neck Surgery,* **pp. 1194–1195)**

338. **(B)** The predisposing factors to this include excessive mucosal destruction, surgery during pharyngitis or purulent sinusitis, revision adenoid surgery with removal of lateral pharyngeal bands, and keloid formation. **(Ref:** *Otolaryngology—Head and Neck Surgery,* **p. 1196)**

339. **(E)** A soft tissue width of more than 7 mm over C2 is pathologic. Widening of the retrotracheal tissue at C6 is considered abnormal in children under 5 years if it is more than 14 mm and in adults if it is more than 22 mm. **(Ref:** *Essential Otolaryngology,* **p. 475)**

340. **(E)** In approximately 50% of deep neck infections, no specific source of infection is found. **(Ref:** *Essential Otolaryngology,* **p. 476)**

26

The Esophagus

341. A 40-year-old male had a large portion of impacted meat removed in the operating room with a rigid esophagoscope. The bronchoscope is at a level of 34 cm from the incisor teeth and the surgeon feels he or she is at the cardia. The average distance from the incisor teeth to the cardia is
    A. 25 cm
    B. 30 cm
    C. 35 cm
    D. 40 cm
    E. 45 cm

342. The lower esophageal sphincter is controlled by an interplay between gastrin and
    A. pepsin
    B. adrenalin
    C. acetylcholine
    D. noradrenalin
    E. serotonin

343. A 50-year-old male is sent for a barium swallow and the report comes back as aperistalsis, esophageal dilatation, and failure of the LES to relax with esophageal retention of ingested material. This patient probably has
   A. scleroderma
   B. presbyesophagus
   C. diffuse esophageal spasm
   D. Barrett esophagitis
   E. achalasia

344. With scleroderma, one usually has a diminished or absent peristalsis in the following segment of the esophagus
   A. upper 1/3
   B. lower 2/3
   C. lower 1/3
   D. midthird
   E. entire esophagus

345. A 30-year-old male has questionable reflux esophagitis. A test that can be done to reproduce his symptoms is
   A. Bernstein test
   B. Smith test
   C. Bougie test
   D. Greisinger test
   E. Frey test

346. The space between the cricopharyngeus and the circular fibers of the esophagus is the
   A. Killian dehiscence space
   B. Lamier–Hacheman space
   C. Zenker space
   D. Killian–Jamieson space
   E. Hacheman space

347. The incidence of hiatus hernia in routine barium swallow in people over the age of 70 is
   A. 30%
   B. 40%
   C. 50%
   D. 60%
   E. 70%

348. A 20-year-old male is suspected of having an esophageal perforation from a foreign body. A test that may be of the most benefit would be
   A. air contrast esophagography
   B. mucosal relief radiography
   C. water-soluble contrast radiography
   D. motion recording radiography
   E. endoscopic ultrasound radiography

349. A 50-year-old male has a Zenker diverticulum on barium swallow. There is an irregularity in the bottom of the pouch. The incidence of carcinoma in a Zenker diverticulum is
   A. 0.3%
   B. 1.0%
   C. 1.5%
   D. 2.2%
   E. 3.0%

350. The endoscopic diathermy method of treating hiatus hernia is called the
   A. Holinger technique
   B. Dohlman technique
   C. Gullane technique
   D. Belsey technique
   E. Sutherland technique

351. The diffuse inflammatory disorder of striated muscle causing symmetric weakness and muscular atrophy with decreased UES pressure is called
   A. scleroderma
   B. muscular dystrophy
   C. dermatomyositis
   D. Barrett disease
   E. Wilms disease

352. A 22-year-old male presents to a hospital emergency department with an abrupt, sharp (knife-like) pain in the epigastrium that began after a sudden vomiting episode. The chest x-ray would probably show
   A. nothing abnormal
   B. right basal pneumonia
   C. left pleural effusion
   D. elevated right diaphragm
   E. bilateral pneumonia

353. A diagnosis of esophageal intramural pseudodiverticulosis is made in a 45-year-old female. The treatment of choice is usually
   A. dilatation of associated strictures
   B. Valium as a muscle relaxant
   C. surgical resection of affected segment of esophagus
   D. the Dohlman technique
   E. oral antibiotics

354. A 40-year-old female patient is diagnosed as having Plummer–Vinson syndrome. Her chances of developing carcinoma of the upper gastrointestinal tract or hypopharynx is approximately
   A. 10%
   B. 20%
   C. 30%
   D. 40%
   E. 50%

355. You make a diagnosis of dysphagia lusoria (Bayford syndrome) in one of your patients. This is due to compression of the esophagus by the anomalous location of
   A. left subclavian artery
   B. right subclavian artery
   C. trachea
   D. right pulmonary artery
   E. left pulmonary artery

The Esophagus

ANSWERS AND DISCUSSION

341. (D) The average distance from the incisor teeth to the cardia in an adult male is 40 cm. In this case, you have probably not reached the cardia and may be in a hiatus hernia pouch. **(Ref:** *Essential Otolaryngology,* **p. 481)**

342. (C) The LES is controlled by gastrin and acetylcholine. In an infant, the angle of entry of the esophagus into the stomach (angle of His) is almost nonexistent so babies reflux readily. **(Ref:** *Essential Otolaryngology,* **p. 481)**

343. (E) Achalasia is a neuromuscular disorder associated with degeneration of ganglion cells of the Auerbach plexus. Esophageal dilatation with failure of the LES to relax for long periods are radiologic hallmarks of this disease. **(Ref:** *Otolaryngology—Head and Neck Surgery,* **pp. 2263–2264)**

344. (B) The lower two thirds of the esophagus are typically involved with scleroderma. There is usually a dilatation of the esophagus on barium swallow and the LES is often patulous. There is a predisposition to esophageal adenocarcinoma. **(Ref:** *Otolaryngology—Head and Neck Surgery,* **p. 2265)**

345. (A) The Bernstein test (acid profusion) is used for definitive diagnosis of reflux esophagitis. Sodium chloride is infused through a levine tube followed by 0.1 N HC1. (**Ref:** *Essential Otolaryngology,* **p. 482**)

346. (B) The Killian dehiscence is between the cricopharyngeus muscle; the Killian–Jamieson space is between the cricopharyngeus and the circular fibers of the esophagus. (**Ref:** *Essential Otolaryngology,* **p. 486**)

347. (E) Approximately 9% of patients under age 40 and 69% over age 70 have a hiatus hernia. (**Ref:** *Essential Otolaryngology,* **pp. 487–488**)

348. (C) Water-soluble contrast radiography is useful if a pharyngeal or esophageal tear is suspected. Barium in the mediastinum may incite an inflammatory reaction but water-soluble contrast media can initiate a terrible pneumonitis or pulmonary edema if aspirated. (**Ref:** *Otolaryngology—Head and Neck Surgery,* **p. 2259**)

349. (A) The incidence of carcinoma in a Zenker diverticulum is approximately 0.3%. The suspicion is raised if blood is seen in the regurgitated material. (**Ref:** *Otolaryngology—Head and Neck Surgery,* **p. 2371**)

350. (B) The Dohlman technique is popular in Europe but less so in North America. There is an increased incidence of mediastinitis using this technique. (**Ref:** *Otolaryngology—Head and Neck Surgery,* **p. 2374**)

351. (C) Dermatomyositis is in contrast to scleroderma as the striated muscles of the hypopharynx and esophagus are involved. (**Ref:** *Essential Otolaryngology,* **p. 488**)

352. (C) Boerhaave syndrome occurs after sudden vomiting. There is usually a 1- to 4-cm tear on the left side of the esophagus, hence the left pleural effusion. (**Ref:** *Essential Otolaryngology,* **p. 490**)

353. (A) About 90% of patients have associated strictures and these should be dilated. Dietary control and antacids offer symptomatic relief. (**Ref:** *Otolaryngology—Head and Neck Surgery,* **pp. 2379–2380)**

354. (E) There is a high incidence (50%) of carcinoma of the upper gastrointestinal tract or hypopharynx in Plummer–Vinson syndrome. About 90% of patients are female and they present with esophageal webs and iron deficiency anemia. (**Ref:** *Essential Otolaryngology,* **p. 492)**

355. (B) Dysphagia lusoria is an uncommon condition of symptomatic compression of the esophagus by the anomalous location of the right subclavian artery (RSA). Normally, the RSA passes posterior to the esophagus in 80% of people, between the trachea and esophagus in 15% of people, and anterior to the trachea and esophagus in 5% of people. (**Ref:** *Essential Otolaryngology,* **p. 494)**

27

Swallowing Disorders

DIRECTIONS (Questions 356 through 365): Each of the numbered items or incomplete statements in this section is followed by answers or completions of the statement. Select the ONE lettered answer or completion that is BEST in each case.

---

356. The oral phase of swallowing can be affected by a lesion in the
   A. hypoglossal canal
   B. foramen ovale
   C. carotid canal
   D. stylomastoid foramen
   E. foramen lacerum

357. A 55-year-old male has no gag reflex on stimulation of the soft palate. The following ganglion is most likely affected
   A. sphenopalatine
   B. ciliary
   C. Meckel
   D. geniculate
   E. Arnold

358. The pharyngeal phase of swallowing is completed by
   A. elevation of the soft palate
   B. a retroflexing epiglottis
   C. closure of the laryngeal aperture

D. cricopharyngeal sphincter relaxation
E. laryngeal elevation

359. A 40-year-old female has dysphagia for liquids and can swallow solids relatively well. This suggests
A. an obstructing tumor
B. a neurologic impairment
C. a tissue deficiency
D. a Zenker diverticulum
E. a stenosis of the esophagus

360. A 50-year-old male presents with what is clinically a globus hystericus. This is associated with a (an)
A. normal physical exam and barium swallow
B. lesion of the upper esophagus
C. stricture of the upper esophagus
D. Zenker diverticulum
E. abnormal direct laryngoscopy

361. Prominence of cricopharyngeal indentation (cricopharyngeal "bar") is regarded as an inconsistent yet frequently observed finding in the following percentage of normal subjects
A. < 5%
B. 10%
C. 15 to 20%
D. 30 to 45%
E. > 50%

362. An anatomic weakness between the cricopharyngeal muscles is called
A. Killian dehiscence
B. Mallory–Weiss syndrome
C. Schatski ring
D. Boerhaave syndrome
E. Ollier syndrome

363. A relative contraindication to cricopharyngeal myotomy is a(n)
- **A.** hiatus hernia with reflux
- **B.** obese patient
- **C.** Zenker diverticulum
- **D.** Schatski ring
- **E.** gastric ulcer

364. A 30-year-old male presents with loss of sensation of the base of the tongue, the pharynx, and the resulting aspiration. This can be associated with a lesion of the
- **A.** foramen lacerum
- **B.** jugular foramen
- **C.** foramen ovale
- **D.** carotid canal
- **E.** stylomastoid foramen

365. The constrictor muscles are supplied by the
- **A.** descending cervicalis nerve
- **B.** ansa hypoglossi nerve
- **C.** descendens hypoglossi nerve
- **D.** accessory nerve
- **E.** vagus nerve

Swallowing Disorders

ANSWERS AND DISCUSSION

356. **(A)** The oral phase of swallowing consists of bolus selection, preparation, control, and delivery. **(Ref:** *Essential Otolaryngology,* **pp. 499–500)**

357. **(A)** The palatine nerves synapse in the sphenopalatine (pterygopatatine) ganglion. **(Ref:** *Otolaryngology—Head and Neck Surgery,* **p. 635)**

358. **(D)** The components of the pharyngeal phase of swallowing include (1) nasopharyngeal closure; (2) bolus advancement by combined action of the base of the tongue and sequenced contraction of the superior, middle, and inferior constrictor muscles; (3) laryngeal elevation by action of the suprahyoid muscles; and (4) closure of the laryngeal aperture by vocal cord adduction and reinforced by the retroflexing epiglottis. **(Ref:** *Essential Otolaryngology,* **pp. 499–500)**

359. **(B)** Generally, dysphagia for solids is associated with a structural abnormality such as an obstructing tumor, tissue deficiency, or stenosis of the food passage. **(Ref:** *Essential Otolaryngology,* **p. 500)**

360. **(A)** Several of these patients may have gastroesophageal reflux and this should be investigated. **(Ref:** *Otolaryngology—Head and Neck Surgery,* **p. 2364)**

361. **(C)** Pooled obstruction of contrast material proximal to the bar and other corroborative examinations such as manometric measurements are helpful in assessing possible cricopharyngeal dysfunction. (**Ref: *Essential Otolaryngology,* p. 503**)

362. **(A)** This is the generally accepted site of herniation of hypopharyngeal diverticula. (**Ref: *Otolaryngology—Head and Neck Surgery,* pp. 2369–2370**)

363. **(A)** Esophageal dyskinesia, reflux, and regurgitation are relative contraindications as reflux gastroesophagitis, combined with an incompetent sphincter, poses risks for laryngotracheal penetration and its consequences. (**Ref: *Essential Otolaryngology,* p. 500**)

364. **(B)** Cranial nerves IX, X, and XI can be affected by any lesion that compromises the jugular foramen. (**Ref: *Otolaryngology–Head and Neck Surgery,* p. 3303**)

365. **(E)** Central lesions or cerebral vascular accidents can cause significant problems related to deglutition. (**Ref: *Essential Otolaryngology,* p. 500**)

28

The Salivary Glands: Benign and Malignant Disease

DIRECTIONS (Questions 366 through 385): Each of the numbered items or incomplete statements in this section is followed by answers or completions of the statement. Select the ONE lettered answer or completion that is BEST in each case.

366. The poststyloid portion of the parapharyngeal space contains the internal jugular vein, internal carotid artery, and cranial nerves
   A. IX, X, and XI
   B. IX, X, XI, and XII
   C. XI and XII
   D. X and XII
   E. IX and X

367. The parotid gland is separated from the submandibular gland by the
   A. stylohyoid
   B. posterior belly of the digastric
   C. mylohyoid
   D. stylomandibular ligament
   E. anterior belly of the digastric

368. When performing a parotidectomy, one has to remember that the mandibular and cervical branches of the facial nerve are intimately associated with the parotid gland and lie in the following position
   A. in the plane of the platysma
   B. directly under the platysma in the plane of the deep cervical fascia
   C. directly over the platysma in the plane of the deep cervical fascia
   D. in the plane of the superficial cervical fascia
   E. very deep under the platysma muscle

369. The parasympathetic nerve supply of the parotid gland synapses in the
   A. otic ganglion
   B. geniculate ganglion
   C. superior salivatory nucleus
   D. spinal cord
   E. superior cervical ganglion

370. In the parotid gland, the following cells produce saliva
   A. myoepithelial cells
   B. intercalated duct cells
   C. excretory duct cells
   D. acinar cells
   E. striated duct cells

371. On radiosialography, this patient with a parotid mass shows focally increased activity. The most likely diagnosis is
   A. mucoepidermoid carcinoma
   B. acinic cell tumor
   C. adenoid cystic carcinoma
   D. squamous cell carcinoma
   E. Warthin tumor

372. A 55-year-old male patient presents with dry mouth and dry eyes. A helpful test in making a diagnosis is
   A. labial biopsy
   B. diagnostic ultrasound

C. sialography
D. CT scan of the parotid gland
E. salivary fluid studies

373. A 30-year-old female has an acutely swollen right parotid gland. The most likely organism to be seen on culture would be
A. Hemophilus influenzae
B. Pseudomonas aeruginosa
C. Bacteroides fragilis
D. Streptococcus pyogenes
E. Staphylococcus aureus

374. In diagnosing a parotid duct stone with plain films, one would be able to see an opaque stone in the following percentage of cases
A. 35%
B. 50%
C. 70%
D. 90%
E. 10%

375. The following test would be helpful in the diagnosis of Sjögren syndome
A. CBC
B. rheumatoid factor
C. liver function tests
D. serum folate
E. serum B_{12}

376. Ten-year-old Frankie has been in direct contact with another child with mumps. If he is going to become infected, one would know in
A. 7 to 14 days
B. < 7 days
C. 14 to 21 days
D. 21 to 30 days
E. > 30 days

377. Patients with mucoepidermoid carcinoma of the salivary gland have a higher risk for development of
   A. liver cancer
   B. colon cancer
   C. renal cancer
   D. lung cancer
   E. breast cancer

378. Malignant oncocytomas of the salivary glands are particularly common in
   A. Hispanics
   B. North American Indians
   C. Eskimos
   D. Orientals
   E. Brazilian Indians

379. This 44-year-old male is diagnosed as having a minor gland adenocarcinoma in the sinonasal region. His most likely occupation would be a
   A. woodworker
   B. heavy metal manufacturer
   C. brew master
   D. coal miner
   E. nuclear power station operator

380. This 60-year-old female is suspected to have a squamous cell carcinoma of the parotid gland. Fine-needle aspiration should give a definitive diagnosis in the following percentage of such cases
   A. < 60%
   B. 60 to 70%
   C. 70 to 80%
   D. 80 to 90%
   E. > 90%

381. This 70-year-old male has a right parotid gland mass with facial nerve paralysis. The most likely diagnosis is
   A. malignant mixed tumors
   B. squamous cell carcinoma
   C. mucoepidermoid carcinoma
   D. adenocarcinoma
   E. adenoid cystic carcinoma

382. The tumor that is thought to arise from the terminal tubules and intercalated duct cells is
  A. malignant mixed tumors
  B. mucoepidermoid carcinoma
  C. adenoid cystic carcinoma
  D. adenocarcinoma
  E. squamous cell carcinoma

383. On this 40-year-old male, fine-needle aspiration of the submandibular gland showed malignant histology. The most likely diagnosis is
  A. adenoid cystic carcinoma
  B. mucoepidermoid carcinoma
  C. adenocarcinoma
  D. squamous cell carcinoma
  E. malignant mixed tumor

384. On histologic exam of this parotid mass, amyloid deposits were seen. The most likely diagnosis is
  A. Warthin tumor
  B. adenoid cystic carcinoma
  C. malignant oncocytoma
  D. carcinoma, *ex.* pleomorphic adenoma
  E. acinic cell carcinoma

385. The highest determinate 5-year survival rate for salivary gland tumors is that of the following tumor
  A. low grade mucoepidermoid
  B. acinic cell
  C. adenoid cystic
  D. adenocarcinoma
  E. malignant mixed

The Salivary Glands: Benign and Malignant Disease

ANSWERS AND DISCUSSION

366. (B) The deep portion of the parotid gland is in contact with the parapharyngeal space. This space contains the styloid process and its three muscles (stylopharyngeus, styloglossus, and stylohyoid). The prestyloid portion contains only muscles and fat. (**Ref:** *Essential Otolaryngology*, **p. 505**)

367. (D) The deep cervical fascia splits to enclose the parotid gland. The anteroinferior portion of this sheet is the stylomandibular ligament. At times, the deep portion of the parotid gland extends between this ligament and the posterior border of the ramus of the mandible into the prestyloid compartment of the parapharyngeal space, forming a parapharyngeal tumor that can be seen and palpated in the oropharynx through the open mouth. (**Ref:** *Essential Otolaryngology*, **p. 505**)

368. (B) This is very important to remember when doing any parotid surgery but also if one is doing any surgical incisions in this area. One must also remember that there can be various common variations of facial nerve branching. (**Ref:** *Otolaryngology—Head and Neck Surgery*, **pp. 1047–1048**)

369. (A) The parasympathetic nerve supply originates in the inferior salivary nucleus (medulla) and travels with the glossopharyngeal nerve and then the Jacobson nerve to the otic ganglion where it synapses. **(Ref: *Essential Otolaryngology*, p. 506)**

370. (D) Secretory cells such as the acinar cells of the parotid gland discharge their products by a process of exocytosis, wherein fusion of secretory granules with a delimited portion of the plasmalemma at the apex of the acinar cell occurs. **(Ref: *Otolaryngology—Head and Neck Surgery*, pp. 989–990)**

371. (E) Warthin tumors concentrate the isotope but do not have a patent duct system and therefore collect the isotope. Rarely, an oncocytoma can mimic this on radiosialography as they have a high mitochondria concentration and consequently increased activity on scans. **(Ref: *Essential Otolaryngology*, p. 511)**

372. (A) A labial biopsy can discriminate between Sjögren syndrome and sarcoidosis. In Sjögren syndrome, there is lymphoid and plasma cell infiltration and acinar atrophy. **(Ref: *Essential Otolaryngology*, pp. 511–512)**

373. (E) The *S. aureus* can be penicillin resistant. Other organisms include *S. pyogenes, S. viridans, S. pneumonococcus,* and *H. influenzae.* **(Ref: *Otolaryngology—Head and Neck Surgery*, p. 1008)**

374. (A) Sialolithiasis preferentially affects the submandibular gland (80% of cases). The calculi are often composed of hydroxyapatite and are multiple in 25% of cases. About 65% of parotid calculi are radiolucent, while 65% of submandibular ones are radiopaque. **(Ref: *Essential Otolaryngology*, pp. 514–515)**

375. (B) Laboratory findings include a positive test for rheumatoid factor, an increased level of serum globulin and C-reactive proteins, and high titers of IgG, IgA, and IgM. Cryoglobulins may also be demonstrated. **(Ref: *Otolaryngology—Head and Neck Surgery*, p. 716)**

376. (C) The duration of the disease is 7 to 10 days. Other organs may be affected, causing orchitis, pancreatitis, nephritis, encephalitis, meningitis, and cochleitis. Antibody titers show a positive S & V antigen titer of more than 1:192. **(Ref: *Essential Otolaryngology*, p. 514)**

377. (E) Mucoepidermoid carcinoma is the most common malignant salivary gland tumor. It arises in the parotid gland (70% of all mucoepidermoid cancers) although it accounts for only 10% of all parotid tumors. **(Ref: *Essential Otolaryngology*, pp. 519–523)**

378. (C) The oncocytomas account for less than 1% of all salivary gland tumors. Most are benign but a small percentage can be malignant. It most commonly occurs in the sixth decade of life. **(Ref: *Otolaryngology—Head and Neck Surgery*, pp. 1034–1035)**

379. (A) Minor salivary gland tumors account for only 15% of all salivary gland tumors. Benign tumors account for 55% of all salivary gland tumors with the most common being pleomorphic adenoma. **(Ref: *Essential Otolaryngology*, p. 525)**

380. (E) Seeding in the needle tracks or facial nerve injury has not been reported in the head and neck, and in fact only two such cases have been reported in any site. **(Ref: *Otolaryngology—Head and Neck Surgery*, p. 1062)**

381. (C) Over 75% of patients with mucoepidermoid carcinoma of the parotid present with an asymptomatic swelling, 13% present with pain, and a small number present with facial nerve paralysis. **(Ref: *Essential Otolaryngology*, p. 522)**

382. (D) Adenocarcinoma accounts for 4% of all parotid tumors and 20% of minor salivary gland tumors. Many varieties of adenocarcinoma have been described (conventional, mucinous, papillary) and they are graded as low, intermediate or high grade. **(Ref: *Essential Otolaryngology*, p. 523)**

383. (A) Adenoid cystic carcinoma is the most common malignant tumor of the submandibular or minor salivary glands. Bone involvement is present in 50% of patients, 25% have facial pain,

20% have facial nerve involvement, and lymphatic metastasis occurs in 15%. (**Ref:** *Essential Otolaryngology,* **p. 523**)

384. (E) Acinic cell carcinoma accounts for only 3% of parotid tumors but almost exclusively occurs in this gland. These tumors are rarely multifocal and 3% are bilateral. (**Ref:** *Essential Otolaryngology,* **p. 523**)

385. (A) Low grade mucoepidermoid carcinoma of the salivary glands has an 84% 15-year survival rate. (**Ref:** *Otolaryngology— Head and Neck Surgery,* **p. 1054**)

29

Carcinoma of the Oral Cavity and Pharynx

DIRECTIONS (Questions 386 through 400): Each of the numbered items or incomplete statements in this section is followed by answers or completions of the statement. Select the ONE lettered answer or completion that is BEST in each case.

---

386. Cancers of the oral cavity and pharynx represent the following percentage of cancers that occur in the United States annually

   A. 1%

   B. 3%

   C. 5%

   D. 10%

   E. 15%

387. A 60-year-old male with carcinoma of the medial portion of the lower lip has metastases to lymph nodes. The nodes that would probably be involved are the

   A. anterior cervical

   B. posterior cervical

   C. submandibular
   D. submental
   E. infraparotid

388. A 65-year-old alcoholic male has a carcinoma in his oral cavity and presents with lymphadenopathy in the upper deep jugular and lateral retropharyngeal nodes. The location of his carcinoma is probably the
   A. lingual aspect of upper gingiva
   B. buccal mucosa
   C. upper lip
   D. lower lip
   E. external canal

389. A 55-year-old female is diagnosed as having carcinoma of the buccal mucosa with regional metastases with no extracapsular spread. Her 5-year survival rate would be approximately
   A. 10 to 20%
   B. 20 to 40%
   C. 50 to 70%
   D. 70 to 80%
   E. 80 to 90%

390. Your patient has a $T_2N_0M_0$ tumor of the oral cavity. This would be stage
   A. 0
   B. I
   C. II
   D. III
   E. IV

391. You have a patient with a stage III carcinoma of the nasopharynx. This would be a
   A. $T_2N_0M_0$
   B. T_yN_0
   C. N_1M_0
   D. $T_3N_0M_0$
   E. T_1N_2

392. You have a patient who has a tumor of the floor of the mouth. His chance of developing another primary cancer of the upper respiratory tract is
  A. 3%
  B. 5%
  C. 10%
  D. 15%
  E. 20%

393. A 70-year-old male presents to your office with a 2-cm lesion on his lower lip that has grown over 3 weeks. It is well circumscribed and has a central keratinized core. The most likely diagnosis is
  A. pyogenic granuloma
  B. squamous cell carcinoma
  C. tuberculous ulcers
  D. necrotizing sialometaplasia
  E. keratoacanthoma

394. A 40-year-old male has a single chronically positive ipsilateral node more than 3 cm but less than 6 cm in diameter. This is a classification of
  A. N_1
  B. N_2
  C. N_{2a}
  D. N_{2b}
  E. N_3

395. A 45-year-old male who is a smoker has a 2-cm pyriform sinus squamous cell carcinoma with no palpable lymph nodes. The incidence of an occult metastasis is approximately
  A. 10%
  B. 18%
  C. 30%
  D. 38%
  E. 45%

396. With carcinoma of the lip, the incidence of upper lip carcinoma is
  A. 5%
  B. 10%

C. 15%
D. 20%
E. 25%

397. A female has a 1-cm squamous cell carcinoma of the lower lip. The chance of her having a neck metastasis is
A. 2%
B. 5 to 10%
C. 10 to 20%
D. 20 to 30%
E. 30 to 40%

398. Squamous cell carcinoma of the hard palate accounts for the following percentage of all upper respiratory tract carcinomas
A. 0.5%
B. 3%
C. 5%
D. 10%
E. 20%

399. Your patient is a 50-year-old male and has a retromolar trigone, squamous cell carcinoma. The chance of this being cervical metastasis is approximately
A. 10%
B. 20%
C. 30%
D. 40%
E. 50%

400. Nasopharyngeal carcinoma in the non-Oriental patient has a bimodal presentation. Of those patients with nasopharyngeal carcinoma, the incidence in under 30 year olds is
A. 5%
B. 10%
C. 15 to 20%
D. 20 to 30%
E. 30 to 40%

Carcinoma of the Oral Cavity and Pharynx

ANSWERS AND DISCUSSION

386. (B) Approximately 3% of all cancers in the United States are located in the oral cavity and pharynx. In India, one half of all cancers are oral and pharyngeal carcinomas. **(Ref:** *Essential Otolaryngology,* **p. 535)**

387. (D) The lateral aspect of the lower lip drains to the submandibular nodes and the medial aspect of the lower lip drains to the submental nodes. **(Ref:** *Otolaryngology—Head and Neck Surgery,* **p. 1250)**

388. (A) Lymphatics of the buccal aspect of the upper and lower alveolar ridges drain to the submental and submandibular lymph nodes. **(Ref:** *Otolaryngology—Head and Neck Surgery,* **pp. 1251–1252)**

389. (C) If extracapsular spread is present, the number of patients who survive for 5 years is reduced to 25 to 30%. Regional metastases are present on initial evaluation in approximately 30% of patients with oral cavity cancer, except for cancers of the lip and hard palate. **(Ref:** *Otolaryngology—Head and Neck Surgery,* **p. 1261)**

390. (C) Stage II is a $T_2N_0M_0$. This means there is a tumor of more than 2 cm but not more than 4 cm in greatest dimension. **(Ref: *Essential Otolaryngology*, p. 538)**

391. (D) Stage III tumor of the oral cavity, oropharynx, nasopharynx, or hypopharynx could be a $T_3N_0M_0$ or $T_1T_2T_3$, N_1, M_0. **(Ref: *Essential Otolaryngology*, pp. 539–540)**

392. (D) Approximately 15% of patients with carcinoma of the oral cavity or any other upper respiratory site will have a synchronous or metachronous tumor. Therefore, it is important to examine other areas as well. **(Ref: *Otolaryngology—Head and Neck Surgery*, p. 1261)**

393. (E) The key here is the rapid growth. These lesions are usually circular with a central crater and may grow rapidly. Pathologically, they can be mistaken for a well-differentiated squamous cell carcinoma. **(Ref: *Otolaryngology—Head and Neck Surgery*, p. 1263)**

394. (C) N_{2a} is a single clinically positive ipsilateral node more than 3 cm and less than 6 cm in diameter. An N_{2b} node is a multiple clinically positive ipsilated node more than 6 cm in diameter. **(Ref: *Otolaryngology—Head and Neck Surgery*, p. 1265)**

395. (D) The chance of an occult metastasis in a pharyngeal site is approximately 38%. The decision is whether to do a neck dissection or irradiate. **(Ref: *Essential Otolaryngology*, pp. 542–543)**

396. (A) About 95% of carcinomas are on the lower lip and only 5% are on the upper lip and commissures. **(Ref: *Essential Otolaryngology*, pp. 543–544)**

397. (B) There is a higher incidence of metastases from the upper lip than the lower lip. The incidence of metastases from the lower lip is less than 10%. **(Ref: *Essential Otolaryngology*, pp. 543–544)**

398. (A) Hard palate carcinomas are rare and only account for 0.5% of all upper respiratory tract carcinomas. **(Ref: *Essential Otolaryngology*, p. 546)**

399. (E) Approximately 50% of patients with a retromolar trigone carcinoma have metastases to their upper deep jugular lymph nodes. (**Ref:** *Essential Otolaryngology,* **pp. 546–547**)

400. (C) Approximately 18% of patients who have SCC of the nasopharynx are under age 30. (**Ref:** *Essential Otolaryngology,* **pp. 549–551**)

30

Cancer of the Larynx, Ear, and Paranasal Sinus

DIRECTIONS (Questions 401 through 415): Each of the numbered items or incomplete statements in this section is followed by answers or completions of the statement. Select the ONE lettered answer or completion that is BEST in each case.

401. The incidence of laryngeal carcinoma is approximately the following percentage of all carcinomas
    A. 0.5%
    B. 2%
    C. 5%
    D. 10%
    E. 15%

402. A 45-year-old male patient is diagnosed on biopsy as having a verrucous carcinoma. The incidence of verrucous carcinoma as a percentage of primary neoplasms of the larynx is
    A. 1%
    B. 2.5%
    C. 3.7%
    D. 5.2%
    E. 7.0%

403. On examination in the operating room, your patient has a frozen section biopsy proven squamous cell carcinoma. The lesion in the supraglottic area appears to involve the cartilage anteriorly. According to TNM staging, this would be classified as a

    A. T_1
    B. T_2
    C. T_3
    D. T_4
    E. T_{4a}

404. By definition, a lesion of the infraglottic area of the larynx has to be at least the following millimeters below the free edge of the vocal cord

    A. 3 mm
    B. 5 mm
    C. 10 mm
    D. 15 mm
    E. 20 mm

405. A 60-year-old male who was diagnosed as having carcinoma of the neck with right neck metastasis asks you what the mortality rate is associated with the actual surgery. You say the risk is

    A. < 1%
    B. 1 to 2%
    C. 2 to 5%
    D. 5 to 10%
    E. 10 to 15%

406. The most important route of spread of supraglottic cancer is

    A. to the anterior cervical lymph nodes
    B. anteriorly into the pre-epiglottic space
    C. superiorly into the base of the tongue
    D. inferiorly into the pyriform sinus
    E. posteriorly into the esophagus

407. A patient presents to your office with hoarseness. On telescopic laryngoscopy, he has fixation of the right vocal cord. You know he has at least a

    A. T_1 lesion
    B. T_2 lesion

    C. T_3 lesion
    D. T_4 lesion
    E. T_{4b} lesion

408. The following percentage of subglottic primary tumors present as T_4 lesions
    A. 10%
    B. 20%
    C. 30%
    D. 45%
    E. 55%

409. According to Sisson, the indication for horizontal supraglottic laryngectomy is normal vocal cord mobility, and the following margin must exist between the inferior border of the tumor and the anterior commissure
    A. 2 mm
    B. 5 mm
    C. 7 mm
    D. 10 mm
    E. 12 mm

410. Early glottic carcinoma $(T_1N_0M_0)$ has an overall cure with radiotherapy and surgical salvage of approximately
    A. 70%
    B. 75%
    C. 80%
    D. 90%
    E. 95%

411. With pyriform sinus carcinoma, the overall survival rate for 3 years is approximately
    A. 10%
    B. 20%
    C. 30%
    D. 40%
    E. 50%

412. One of the unusual symptoms of carcinoma of the ear canal as compared to most other sites of carcinoma is
    A. hearing loss
    B. bleeding
    C. pain
    D. infection
    E. nerve paralysis

413. A 45-year-old male patient has a positive biopsy of an adenocarcinoma of the right ethmoid sinus. In the patient's social history, you may find his occupation is a
    A. woodworker
    B. heavy metal worker
    C. fireman
    D. farmer
    E. nuclear power plant employee

414. Your patient has a squamous cell carcinoma of the right maxillary antrum with invasion of the cheek. This is at least a
    A. T_1
    B. T_2
    C. T_3
    D. T_4
    E. T_x

415. The 5-year survival rate of squamous cell carcinoma of the ethmoid sinus with metastases is
    A. 50%
    B. 40%
    C. 20%
    D. 10%
    E. 0%

Cancer of the Larynx, Ear, and Paranasal Sinus

ANSWERS AND DISCUSSION

401. (B) Cancer of the larynx represents less than 2% of all carcinomas. In the United States, there are approximately 10,900 new patients with laryngeal carcinoma annually. (**Ref:** *Essential Otolaryngology,* **p. 555**)

402. (C) Verrucous carcinoma occurs in 3.7% of primary carcinomas of the larynx. (**Ref:** *Essential Otolaryngology,* **p. 560**)

403. (D) A T_4 lesion is a tumor in which the lesion has invaded cartilage or tissue beyond the larynx. (**Ref:** *Otolaryngology—Head and Neck Surgery,* **p. 1930**)

404. (C) An infraglottic lesion arises 10 mm below the free edge of the vocal cord to the inferior border of the cricoid cartilage. (**Ref:** *Essential Otolaryngology,* **p. 563**)

405. (C) The mortality rate associated with laryngectomy with radical neck dissection is 2 to 5%. The mortality rate goes up to 8.5% when preoperative radiotherapy is given. (**Ref:** *Essential Otolaryngology,* **pp. 566–567**)

406. (B) Spread of supraglottic cancer anteriorly into the pre-epiglottic space occurs by means of fenestrae in the elastic cartilage of the epiglottis through which cancer may spread. (**Ref:** *Otolaryngology—Head and Neck Surgery,* **p. 1933)**

407. (C) Fixation of the vocal cord automatically means that it is a T_3 lesion. The principal mechanism of vocal cord fixation has been identified as replacement of the thyroarytenoid muscle. (**Ref:** *Otolaryngology—Head and Neck Surgery,* **p. 1934)**

408. (D) Primary subglottic tumors are rare and silent. Approximately 45% present as T_4 lesions. (**Ref:** *Otolaryngology—Head and Neck Surgery,* **p. 1935)**

409. (C) A margin of 5 mm must exist between the inferior border of the tumor and the interior commissure. There are numerous other criteria for horizontal supraglottic laryngectomy including normal pulmonary function. (**Ref:** *Essential Otolaryngology,* **p. 563)**

410. (E) Approximately 96.1% in a series of 1700 patients with early glottic carcinoma had an overall cure rate. (**Ref:** *Essential Otolaryngology,* **p. 566)**

411. (D) This tends to be a very aggressive tumor with a low overall cure rate. (**Ref:** *Essential Otolaryngology,* **p. 566)**

412. (C) In 50% of patients with squamous cell carcinoma of the external canal, there is intense pain that is out of proportion to the pathologic and clinical findings. (**Ref:** *Essential Otolaryngology,* **p. 573)**

413. (A) Woodworkers have an increased incidence of adenocarcinoma of the ethmoids, while heavy metal workers have an increased risk for paranasal sinus squamous cell cancer. (**Ref:** *Essential Otolaryngology,* **p. 568)**

414. (C) A T_3 tumor is a more extensive tumor invading the cheek, orbit, anterior ethmoid sinus, or pterygoid muscle. (**Ref:** *Essential Otolaryngology,* **p. 570)**

415. (E) This is a very aggressive tumor with extremely poor survival. (**Ref:** *Essential Otolaryngology,* **pp. 571–572)**

31

Thyroid and Parathyroid Glands

DIRECTIONS (Questions 416 through 425): Each of the numbered items or incomplete statements in this section is followed by answers or completions of the statement. Select the ONE lettered answer or completion that is BEST in each case.

416. During thyroid surgery, the external branch of the superior laryngeal nerve is severed. This branch innervates the
   A. cricothyroid muscle
   B. interarytenoid muscle—transverse
   C. vocalis muscle
   D. interarytenoid muscle—oblique
   E. thyroartenoid muscle

417. A 20-year-old patient presents with an anterior neck swelling over the hyoid bone in the midline. You suspect a thyroglossal duct cyst. In anatomic specimens, there are remnants of thyroglossal duct cysts in the following percentage of patients
   A. 2%
   B. 7%
   C. 13%
   D. 20%
   E. 25%

418. The following percentage of T_4 is bound to TBG in the blood
    A. 15%
    B. 5%
    C. 60%
    D. 30%
    E. 80%

419. A 50-year-old male had a thyroidectomy for differentiated carcinoma of the thyroid. A blood test that is helpful to monitor his tumor would be
    A. serum thyroglobulin
    B. serum T_4
    C. serum T_3
    D. serum TSH
    E. serum TBC

420. A 40-year-old male has been feeling tired and collapses into a myxedema coma. He has hypothermia, cardiovascular collapse, hypoventilation, and coma. Blood work shows
    A. Na^+, serum glucose, and lactic acidosis
    B. Na^+ and serum glucose
    C. hyponatremia, hypoglycemia, and lactic acidosis
    D. lactic acidosis and Na^+
    E. lactic acidosis and serum glucose

421. A 30-year-old female presents to your office with extreme symptoms of fatigue that have persisted over 6 months. Blood tests reveal normal T_4, T_3RU, FT_4I, T_3, and elevated TSH. You suspect
    A. tertiary hypothyroidism
    B. secondary hypothyroidism
    C. primary occult hypothyroidism
    D. primary overt hypothyroidism
    E. euthyroidism

422. A 70-year-old male is hospitalized in the ICU with severe pneumonia and congestive heart failure. An accurate screening for hypothyroidism would be
    A. TSH IMA alone
    B. TSH IMA and free T_4

C. TRH alone
D. T$_3$RU
E. T$_4$ alone

423. A 30-year-old male is diagnosed as having Graves disease. A frequently used medication that blocks peripheral conversion of T$_4$ to T$_3$ is
  A. propylthiouracil
  B. methimazole
  C. propanolol
  D. betamethasone
  E. digoxin

424. A 40-year-old female had a sudden onset of a flu-like disease, myalgia, temperature of 102°, and neck pain radiating to the ear. Her ESR was 120 and she had a low RAIU. Treatment would be
  A. antibiotics
  B. propylthiouracil
  C. methimazole
  D. analgesics and beta blockers
  E. monovalent cations

425. Medullary carcinoma, pheochromocytoma, and parathyroid hyperplasia is classified as
  A. MTC with MEN II A
  B. MTC with MEN II B
  C. familial non-MEN MTC
  D. sporadic MTC
  E. MTC

Thyroid and Parathyroid Glands

ANSWERS AND DISCUSSION

416. **(A)** The superior laryngeal nerve innervates the cricothyroid muscle, which tenses the vocal cord. During thyroid surgery, one should avoid this. **(Ref:** *Essential Otolaryngology,* **p. 581)**

417. **(B)** Ellis and Van Nostrand (1977) found remnants of the thyroglossal duct in 7% of specimens. **(Ref:** *Otolaryngology—Head and Neck Surgery,* **p. 2403)**

418. **(E)** About 80% of T_4 is bound to TBG, 15% to thyroid-binding prealbumin (TBPA), and the remainder to serum albumin. **(Ref:** *Essential Otolaryngology,* **p. 583)**

419. **(A)** Thyroglobulin is a tumor marker for differentiated thyroid carcinoma. A progressively increasing serum TG is an indication of tumor progression. **(Ref:** *Essential Otolaryngology,* **p. 586)**

420. **(C)** Metabolic derangements in myxedema coma include hyponatremia, hypoglycemia, and lactic acidosis. The mortality rate is as high as 50%. **(Ref:** *Essential Otolaryngology,* **pp. 588–589)**

421. **(C)** This is the pattern in primary occult hypothyroidism. The TRH is also excessive on testing. **(Ref:** *Otolaryngology—Head and Neck Surgery,* **p. 2421)**

198

422. (B) Most experts agree that the best screening test for hypothyroidism in ambulatory patients is a TSH IMA alone and for hospitalized patients a combination of TSH IMA and a test to estimate free T_4. (**Ref:** *Otolaryngology—Head and Neck Surgery,* **p. 2421**)

423. (A) Propylthiouracil blocks peripheral conversion of T_4 to T_3. One must monitor the patient closely for bone marrow suppression, which is usually reversible if detected early. (**Ref:** *Essential Otolaryngology,* **p. 590**)

424. (D) She has pseudogranulomatous or de Quervain thyroiditis. In severe cases, a short course of steroids is necessary. The disease usually lasts 2 to 5 months. (**Ref:** *Otolaryngology—Head and Neck Surgery,* **pp. 2429–2430**)

425. (A) This is MTC with MEN II A and the most useful blood test is serum calcitonin. (**Ref:** *Essential Otolaryngology,* **p. 593**)

32

Carotid Body Tumor, Hemangioma, Lymphangioma, Melanoma, Cysts, and Tumors of the Jaw

---

DIRECTIONS (Questions 426 through 435): Each of the numbered items or incomplete statements in this section is followed by answers or completions of the statement. Select the ONE lettered answer or completion that is BEST in each case.

---

426. A 45-year-old male is diagnosed as having a carotid body tumor. He asks you what the incidence of mortality is if you have to sacrifice the carotid artery. You say it is

    A. 5%

    B. 10 to 20%

    C. 20 to 30%

    D. 30 to 50%

    E. > 60%

427. The following percent of carotid body tumors can be malignant
   A. < 2%
   B. 5 to 10%
   C. 10 to 20%
   D. 20 to 30%
   E. 30 to 40%

428. The most common site of deep hemangiomas within the head and neck are within the
   A. omohyoid space
   B. masseter muscles
   C. submandibular space
   D. lower neck
   E. submental space

429. The incidence of hemangiomas at age 1 year in full-term white infants is
   A. 2%
   B. 3 to 5%
   C. 5 to 8%
   D. 10 to 12%
   E. > 15%

430. Kasabach–Merritt syndrome is an abnormality in which one would find on hematologic testing
   A. decreased platelets
   B. increased BUN, Cr
   C. increased Na^+, decreased Cl^-
   D. increased LFTs (liver function test)
   E. increased TSH

431. This 50-year-old female presents with a 1-cm lesion in the left nares. The diagnosis is made on biopsy of a hemangiopericytoma. The incidence of metastasis is usually
   A. < 2%
   B. 5 to 10%
   C. 10 to 20%
   D. 20 to 30%
   E. > 35%

432. A 7-year-old female has a dome-shaped lesion on her cheek that is pink in color and measures about 1 cm in diameter. Biopsy is benign. The diagnosis is
   A. Spitz nevus
   B. halo nevus
   C. blue nevus
   D. compound nevus
   E. intradermal nevus

433. A 40-year-old male patient of yours has a skin biopsy done that shows malignant melanoma. It is a Clarke III. Its depth of penetration is
   A. 0.25 mm
   B. 0.25 to 0.5 mm
   C. 0.5 to 0.75 mm
   D. 0.75 to 1.5 mm
   E. 1.5 to 2.0 mm

434. A 45-year-old female patient has an area of dark oral pigmentation. She also has intestinal polyposis. The most probable diagnosis is
   A. melanoma
   B. Peutz–Jeghers syndrome
   C. Cooley anemia
   D. pellagra
   E. sprue

435. Cysts that form from the enamel organ before any dental tissue develops are called
   A. radicular
   B. dentigenous cysts
   C. eruption cysts
   D. primordial cysts
   E. odontogenic keratocysts

Carotid Body Tumor, Hemangioma, Lymphangioma, Melanoma, Cysts, and Tumors of the Jaw

ANSWERS AND DISCUSSION

426. (D) Sacrificing the internal carotid artery without applying a graft carries a 30 to 50% mortality with another 40% incidence of neurologic deficits. (**Ref:** *Essential Otolaryngology,* p. 612)

427. (B) Approximately 5 to 10% of these tumors can be malignant. (**Ref:** *Essential Otolaryngology,* p. 612)

428. (B) The highest incidence of deep hemangiomas is within the masseter muscles. (**Ref:** *Essential Otolaryngology,* p. 613)

429. (D) Hemangioma is the most common tumor of infancy. The majority appear in the first 6 months of life. Eighty percent are solitary, whereas 20% are multiple. (**Ref:** *Otolaryngology—Head and Neck Surgery,* p. 336)

430. (A) Kasabach–Merritt syndrome or platelet trapping coagulopathy is a hematologic complication of hemangioma that can be life threatening. There are decreased platelets and increased PT, PTT. (**Ref:** *Otolaryngology—Head and Neck Surgery,* **p. 338**)

431. (E) The cell of origin in hemangiopericytoma is the capillary pericyte of Zimmerman. These are very malignant tumors. Wide excision is the treatment of choice. (**Ref:** *Essential Otolaryngology,* **p. 617**)

432. (A) Spitz nevi occur in children and nothing need be done further with these after diagnosis is made. (**Ref:** *Essential Otolaryngology,* **p. 569**)

433. (D) Clarke levels I and II lesions are less than 0.75 mm. Clarke level III is 0.75 to 1.5 mm and Clarke levels IV and V are greater than 1.5 mm. (**Ref:** *Otolaryngology—Head and Neck Surgery,* **p. 425**)

434. (B) Peutz–Jeghers syndrome can have oral pigmentation and polyposis. The oral lesions have to be differentiated from melanoma of the mucous membrane. (**Ref:** *Essential Otolaryngology,* **p. 621**)

435. (D) Primordial cysts form from the enamel organ before any dental tissue develops. They usually occur in the mandibular third molar. (**Ref:** *Essential Otolaryngology,* **p. 626**)

33

Infections of the Ear

DIRECTIONS (Questions 436 through 450): Each of the numbered items or incomplete statements in this section is followed by answers or completions of the statement. Select the ONE lettered answer or completion that is BEST in each case.

---

436. The two most common pathogens isolated from the middle ear fluid of an otitis media are *H. influenzae* and

- **A.** *Staphylococcus aureus*
- **B.** *Streptococcus pneumoniae*
- **C.** *Branhamella catarrhalis*
- **D.** *Streptococcus,* group A
- **E.** mixed

437. In epidemiologic studies, the following percentage of children have had at least one episode of otitis media

- **A.** 40%
- **B.** 50%
- **C.** 60%
- **D.** 70%
- **E.** > 80%

438. The overall complication rate from PE tubes is approximately
   A. 1%
   B. 5%
   C. 10%
   D. 20%
   E. 30%

439. A 3-year-old female has had myringotomies and tubes. Her mother asks you what are the chances that she will not require further tube insertion. You tell her that the chance of not requiring further surgery is
   A. 60%
   B. 70%
   C. 80%
   D. 90%
   E. > 90%

440. A 4-year-old male who has measles presents to your office with a large tympanic membrane perforation, foul-smelling otorrhea, and sloughing of the annulus tympanicus. The probable organism that would be isolated on culture and sensitivity would be
   A. *Pseudomonas aeruginosa*
   B. *S. pneumoniae*
   C. *B. hemolytic streptococcus*
   D. *S. aureus*
   E. *B. catarrhalis*

441. The most common organism isolated in acute mastoiditis is
   A. *S. pneumoniae*
   B. *Strep. pyogenes*
   C. *S. aureus*
   D. *Pseudomonas aeruginosa*
   E. *B. catarrhalis*

442. The incidence of postoperative hemorrhage after adenoidectomy is
   A. < 0.5%
   B. 1 to 2%
   C. 3 to 5%
   D. 5 to 10%
   E. > 10%

443. The most common organism isolated in chronic suppurative otitis media with perforation is
A. *Bacteroides fragilis*
B. *Pseudomonas aeruginosa*
C. *H. influenzae*
D. *B. catarrhalis*
E. *S. aureus*

444. A 45-year-old immune-suppressed AIDS patient presents with a painless draining ear. The discharge is scanty, thin, and odorless. There is a tympanic membrane perforation with pale granulations. The patient has a hearing loss out of proportion to other symptoms. The most likely diagnosis is
A. acute necrotizing otitis media
B. tuberculosis otitis media
C. syphilitic otitis media
D. bullous myringitis
E. herpes zoster oticus

445. Sadé and Berw described four states of tympanic membrane retraction. Stage II is
A. retracted tympanic membrane
B. adhesive otitis media
C. retraction with perforation
D. middle ear atelectasis
E. retraction with contact onto the incus

446. The theory of cholesteatoma formation in which retraction pockets of the pars flaccida deepen because of negative middle ear pressure and as the retraction pocket deepens the desquamated keratin cannot be cleared is called the
A. invagination theory
B. epithelial invasion theory
C. basal cell hyperplasia theory
D. metaplasia of the middle ear epithelium theory
E. funnel theory

447. The most common anaerobic organism in chronic otitis media with discharge is
   A. *Fusobacterium* spp
   B. *Clostridium bacteroides* spp
   C. *Eubacterium* spp
   D. *Peptococcus*
   E. *Propionibacterium acnes*

448. In chronic otitis media without cholesteatomas, osteitis was present in
   A. 20%
   B. 40%
   C. 60%
   D. 70%
   E. 90%

449. According to Wullstein, after tympanomastoidectomy in which the surgeon reconstructs a new eardrum on top of an upright, freely mobile stapes, it is called
   A. type I
   B. type II
   C. type III
   D. type IV
   E. type V

450. A fistula test will be present in the following percentage of patients with a labyrinthine fistula
   A. 33%
   B. 40%
   C. 66%
   D. 85%
   E. 100%

Infections of the Ear

ANSWERS AND DISCUSSION

436. (B) *Streptococcus pneumoniae* is the most common organism isolated from effusions of otitis media. (**Ref:** *Essential Otolaryngology*, **p. 637**)

437. (E) Greater than 80% of children will have had at least one episode of otitis media. (**Ref:** *Otolaryngology—Head and Neck Surgery*, **p. 2809**)

438. (C) The overall complication rate is approximately 10% after having PE tubes inserted. (**Ref:** *Essential Otolaryngology*, **p. 640**)

439. (C) Approximately 80% of children will respond with one insertion of PE tubes. (**Ref:** *Essential Otolaryngology*, **p. 640**)

440. (C) Acute necrotizing otitis media is a virulent form of acute otitis media. The pathologic process is a true necrosis of the soft tissues and the bones of the middle ear and the mastoid. (**Ref:** *Essential Otolaryngology*, **p. 638**)

441. (A) *S. pneumoniae* is the most common organism isolated from *S. pyogenes* and *S. aureus*. (**Ref:** *Essential Otolaryngology*, **pp. 638–639**)

442. (A) The incidence of bleeding after adenoidectomy is approximately 0.4%. **(Ref:** *Otolaryngology—Head and Neck Surgery,* **p. 2820)**

443. (B) In chronic otitis media, the organisms are much different than in acute otitis media. The most common organism isolated is *Pseudomonas aeruginosa.* **(Ref:** *Essential Otolaryngology,* **p. 641)**

444. (B) This probably represents tuberculous otitis media. Diagnosis is made from direct smears, cultures, and histologic examination of granulation tissue removed from the middle ear or mastoid. Isoniazid and para-aminosalicylic acid (PAS) is commonly used for initial treatment. **(Ref:** *Essential Otolaryngology,* **pp. 641–642)**

445. (E) Stage III is middle ear atelectasis, stage IV is adhesive otitis media, and stage I is retracted tympanic membrane. **(Ref:** *Otolaryngology—Head and Neck Surgery,* **p. 2825)**

446. (A) The invagination theory of cholesteatoma formation is regarded as one of the primary mechanisms for formulation of attic cholesteatoma. **(Ref:** *Otolaryngology—Head and Neck Surgery,* **pp. 2826–2828)**

447. (B) Significant anaerobic bacteria are present in chronic otitis media. *C. bacteroides* is the most common anaerobic bacteria present. **(Ref:** *Otolaryngology—Head and Neck Surgery,* **p. 2828)**

448. (E) Meyerhoff et al (1978) found osteitis in 90.2%, mucoperiosteal fibrosis in 76.4%, granulation tissue in 69.1%, tympanosclerosis in 27.6%, and cholesterol granuloma in 13%. The above was in ears with chronic otitis media without cholesteatoma. **(Ref:** *Otolaryngology—Head and Neck Surgery,* **p. 2829)**

449. (C) This is a type III reconstruction. (**Ref:** *Essential Otolaryngology,* **pp. 646–648**)

450. (C) The fistula test produces vertigo and deviation of the eyes in the application of pressure to the affected ear. A positive fistula test is present in two thirds of the cases with a labyrinthine fistula. (**Ref:** *Essential Otolaryngology,* **pp. 652–663**)

34

Noninfectious Diseases
of the Ear

DIRECTIONS (Questions 451 through 465): Each of the numbered items or incomplete statements in this section is followed by answers or completions of the statement. Select the ONE lettered answer or completion that is BEST in each case.

451. The percentage of patients with otosclerosis with a positive family history is
- **A.** 20%
- **B.** 30%
- **C.** 40%
- **D.** 50%
- **E.** 60%

452. The audiogram on page 213 is consistent with
- **A.** tympanic membrane perforation
- **B.** middle ear trauma
- **C.** early mild otosclerosis
- **D.** serous otitis media
- **E.** chronic otitis media

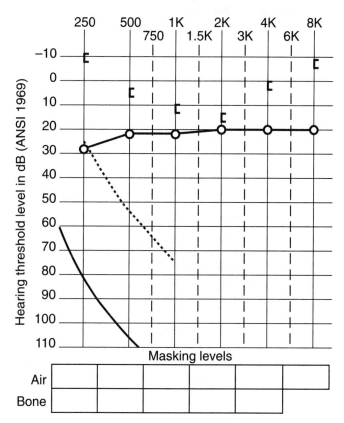

LEFT EAR
Frequency in Hertz

453. One of the main differences histologically between Paget disease and otosclerosis is
A. the stapedial muscle is involved in Paget disease
B. the periosteal and endochondrial layers are involved in Paget disease
C. the periosteal layer is mainly involved in Paget disease
D. all three layers are involved in Paget disease
E. the footplate and ossicles are involved in Paget disease

454. During stapedectomy, there is a luxation of the incus. This usually results in
  A. aborting the operation
  B. trying to fix the incus back into place
  C. using a malleus–oval window prosthesis
  D. removing all ossicles and layering the tympanic membrane over the oval window
  E. using the malleus as the prosthesis anchor

455. During stapedectomy, a segment of footplate enters the vestibule and is seen deep in the vestibule. One should
  A. not go after it but proceed in the usual manner
  B. use a 3-mm hook to attempt to remove it
  C. use a very small number 20 suction
  D. abort the surgery
  E. do a 0.5-mm burr hole and remove the segment

456. In bilateral otosclerosis, it is appropriate to
  A. wait 1 year between surgeries
  B. do both ears at the same time
  C. wait 2 to 3 months between surgeries
  D. not do the second ear under any circumstances
  E. do the second ear if the first surgery was not successful

457. A 40-year-old female did well after stapedectomy for 6 months then presented with a 60-dB hearing loss. The most likely diagnosis is
  A. advanced otosclerosis
  B. granuloma formation
  C. perilymph fistula
  D. incus necrosis
  E. loose wire

458. The incidence of granuloma after stapedectomy is
  A. 1 to 2%
  B. 5%
  C. 10%
  D. 15%
  E. 20%

459. With sudden hearing loss, the following percent have a spontaneous return of normal hearing
   A. < 2%
   B. 10%
   C. 20%
   D. 30%
   E. 60%

460. A 28-year-old male presents to your office with a diagnosed glomus jugulare tumor of the middle ear. There is facial paralysis and a sensorineural loss. Radiographs show enlargement of the jugular foramen but no bone erosion. According to Alford and Gilford, this is termed a
   A. stage 0
   B. stage I
   C. stage II
   D. stage III
   E. stage IV

461. Routine autopsies reveal an incidence of acoustic neuroma of
   A. 0.05%
   B. 0.5%
   C. 2%
   D. 5%
   E. 10%

462. A 40-year-old male is diagnosed as having an acoustic neuroma. The brainstem evoked response audiometry would be expected to show an intra-auricular latency of
   A. < 0.1 milliseconds
   B. 0.1 to 0.2 milliseconds
   C. 0.2 to 0.3 milliseconds
   D. 0.3 to 0.4 milliseconds
   E. > 0.4 milliseconds

463. A 1-year-old male presented with fever, splenomegaly, hepatomegaly, lymphadenopathy, skeletal lesions, and anemia. He died in 10 days. The most probable diagnosis is
    A. Letterer–Siwe disease
    B. Hand–Schuller–Christian disease
    C. eosinophilic granuloma
    D. fibrous dysplasia
    E. childhood sarcoidosis

464. A 14-year-old female presents with painless swelling of the right cheek. Radiographic appearance shows a typical loss of cellular structure and increased radiolucency due to replacement of osseous substance by fibrous tissue. The most probable diagnosis is
    A. Paget disease
    B. Hand–Schuller–Christian disease
    C. Ollier enchondromatosis
    D. fibrous dysplasia
    E. hyperthyroidism

465. A 15-year-old male presents with radiologic lesion of the mastoid cortex with involvement of the facial nerve and jugular foramen involvement. Also, he has exophthalmos and diabetes insipidus. The most probable diagnosis is
    A. Letterer–Siwe disease
    B. Hand–Schuller–Christian disease
    C. fibrous dysplasia
    D. Ollier enchondromatosis
    E. Paget disease

Noninfectious Diseases of the Ear

ANSWERS AND DISCUSSION

451. **(E)**   Otosclerosis has a 60% incidence of positive family history. **(Ref:** *Essential Otolaryngology,* **p. 685)**

452. **(C)**   This is typical of the classic Carhart notch seen in otosclerosis. **(Ref:** *Otolaryngology—Head and Neck Surgery,* **p. 3000)**

453. **(C)**   In osteitis deformans or Paget disease, the periosteal layer is mainly involved and there is diffuse involvement of the temporal bone. **(Ref:** *Essential Otolaryngology,* **pp. 685–686)**

454. **(C)**   There is complete disruption of the incudomalleal joint, which means that the incus be removed and a malleus-oval window prosthesis be used. **(Ref:** *Essential Otolaryngology,* **pp. 687–688)**

455. **(A)**   Every effort must be made to avoid this but if it occurs one should carry on and complete the operation. These patients usually experience postoperative vertigo for several weeks and unsteadiness for months. **(Ref:** *Essential Otolaryngology,* **p. 689)**

456. **(A)**   One must be careful in doing a second ear. The second ear should only be attempted if the first ear is very successful and the hearing remains stable for a year with no vestibular or sensorineural hearing problems. (**Ref:** *Otolaryngology—Head and Neck Surgery,* **p. 3009**)

457. (**D**) The most common cause of this is incus necrosis. A repeat procedure is necessary and a Steffan procedure (drilling a notch in the long process to receive the wire) or using a stainless steel bucket prosthesis may be required. (**Ref:** *Otolaryngology—Head and Neck Surgery,* **p. 3013**)

458. (**A**) Approximately 1 to 2% of cases of stapedectomy may result in reparative granuloma. There is usually a progressive sensorineural hearing loss with marked loss of speech discrimination. Emergency surgical intervention is imperative. (**Ref:** *Essential Otolaryngology,* **p. 690**)

459. (**D**) Approximately one third of patients have a return to normal hearing, one third are left with a 40- to 60-dB speech reception threshold, and one third have total loss of useful hearing. (**Ref:** *Essential Otolaryngology,* **p. 700**)

460. (**C**) This is a stage II according to Alford and Gilford. Stage III has multiple cranial nerve involvement and in stage IV there is intracranial extension. (**Ref:** *Essential Otolaryngology,* **pp. 702–703**)

461. (**C**) Routine autopsies revealed an incidence of 2.4% of asymptomatic acoustic neuroma. (**Ref:** *Essential Otolaryngology,* **p. 704**)

462. (**E**) Intra-aural latency is usually less than 0.2 milliseconds and is found to be 0.4 milliseconds or more in acoustic neuromas. (**Ref:** *Essential Otolaryngology,* **p. 705**)

463. (**A**) Letterer–Siwe is a rare, rapidly fatal form of acute desseminated histocytosis that occurs in children before age 2 years. (**Ref:** *Essential Otolaryngology,* **p. 1101**)

464. (**D**) This is a typical pattern of fibrous dysplasia and treatment is by surgical excision. (**Ref:** *Essential Otolaryngology,* **p. 1117**)

465. (**B**) This is a classic example of Hand–Schuller–Christian disease. Treatment involves irradiation. The mortality rate is 30%. (**Ref:** *Essential Otolaryngology,* **pp. 1101–1102**)

35

The Nose and Sinuses

DIRECTIONS (Questions 466 through 485): Each of the numbered items or incomplete statements in this section is followed by answers or completions of the statement. Select the ONE lettered answer or completion that is BEST in each case.

---

466. The nasolacrimal duct opens at the level of the
- **A.** middle meatus
- **B.** superior meatus
- **C.** inferior meatus
- **D.** sphenoethmoid recess
- **E.** supreme meatus

467. The arterial blood supply of the anteriosuperior portion of the septum and lateral wall is from the
- **A.** descending palatine
- **B.** anterior ethmoidal artery
- **C.** posterior ethmoidal artery
- **D.** sphenopalatine
- **E.** pharyngeal

468. The Kiesselbach plexus in the Little area is formed by the superior labial artery and the
   A. pharyngeal artery
   B. posterior ethmoid
   C. anterior ethmoid
   D. descending palatine
   E. sphenopalatine

469. The average adult nose produces the following amount of secretions per day
   A. 500 mL
   B. 250 mL
   C. 1000 mL
   D. 2000 mL
   E. 4000 mL

470. A 30-year-old male has an acute furunculosis of the nose. The most likely infecting organism is
   A. *Staphylococcus aureus*
   B. *Streptococcus pyogenes*
   C. *Pseudomonas aeruginosa*
   D. *Escherichia coli*
   E. *Candida albicans*

471. The most commonly fractured site in the body is the
   A. finger
   B. leg
   C. arm
   D. cheek
   E. nose

472. A young adult male is in a motor vehicle accident and has sustained facial trauma. He still has copious clear watery drainage from his nose 24 hours later. The next step is
   A. placing him on prophylactic antibiotics
   B. bilateral nasal packing
   C. testing for glucose in secretions
   D. intrathecal injection of fluorescein with pledgets in the nose
   E. observation

473. The Keisselbach plexus accounts for the following percentage of epistaxis
    A. 50%
    B. 60%
    C. 70%
    D. 80%
    E. 90%

474. Angiography with Gelfoam embolization of the sphenopalatine artery branches may be necessary to control severe bleeding from the
    A. anterior superior septal wall
    B. anterior septal wall
    C. posterior septal wall
    D. lateral posterior wall
    E. tonsillar bed

475. In children with choanal atresia, the following percentage is of membranous origin
    A. 90%
    B. 70%
    C. 50%
    D. 10%
    E. 30%

476. Initially, bilateral choanal atresia is treated with
    A. immediate emergency surgery
    B. McGovern nipple
    C. nasal catheters
    D. placing a child on his or her abdomen
    E. observation

477. A nasal smear showing mastocytosis with sparsity of eosinophils is typical of
    A. allergic rhinitis
    B. rhinitis medicamentosa
    C. eosinophilic nonallergic rhinitis
    D. vasomotor rhinitis
    E. atrophic rhinitis

478. In establishing the diagnosis of Wegener granulomatosis, one of the following tests is most helpful
   A. stool for occult blood
   B. PT, PTT, platelets
   C. CBC
   D. liver function tests
   E. urinalysis

479. A 50-year-old male has lymphoepithelioma of the nasopharynx. The treatment of choice is
   A. radical surgery
   B. chemotherapy
   C. no therapy—unresponsive to treatment
   D. radiotherapy
   E. a combination of surgery and chemotherapy

480. One of the side effects of streptomycin may be
   A. hyperosmia
   B. hyposmia
   C. anosmia
   D. no effect on sense of smell
   E. parosmia

481. This 55-year-old male was diagnosed as having inverted papilloma of the nose. You can tell him that it may develop into squamous cell carcinoma in the following percentage of cases
   A. 10%
   B. 30%
   C. 50%
   D. 20%
   E. 40%

482. The major landmark in intranasal ethmoidectomy to identify the cribiform plate is the
   A. attachment of the superior turbinate
   B. attachment of the inferior turbinate
   C. middle meatus
   D. inferior meatus
   E. superior attachment of the middle turbinate

483. In a debilitated patient, with sinusitis in which the sinus x-rays show a radiation-dense shadow resembling a metallic foreign body, the most likely organism to grow on C & S would be
  A. aspergillosis
  B. mucormycosis
  C. *Streptococcus pyogenes*
  D. *Hemophilus influenzae*
  E. *Staphylococcus aureus*

484. The most common malignant tumor of the paranasal sinuses is
  A. adenocarcinoma
  B. transitional cell carcinoma
  C. malignant melanoma
  D. squamous cell carcinoma
  E. adenoid cystic carcinoma

485. A doughy swelling of the skin over the frontal sinuses in an individual with a frontal sinus infection is called
  A. Felty syndrome
  B. Brown tumor
  C. Pott puffy tumor
  D. Hallgren tumor
  E. Seckel tumor

The Nose and Sinuses

ANSWERS AND DISCUSSION

466. (C) Damage to the nasolacrimal duct can occur during endoscopic sinus surgery. The orifice of the duct is located on the lateral wall 3.0 to 3.5 cm behind the posterior margin of the nostril. **(Ref: *Essential Otolaryngology*, p. 716)**

467. (B) The anterior ethmoidal artery, along with branches from the sphenopalatine, greater palatine, and superior labial, form the Little area on the septum. **(Ref: *Otolaryngology—Head and Neck Surgery*, p. 632)**

468. (E) This is the most common site of epistaxis in the nose. **(Ref: *Otolaryngology—Head and Neck Surgery*, p. 633)**

469. (C) Mucus contains muramidase, which breaks down bacterial cell walls, as well as immunoglobulins A and E (IgA, IgE). **(Ref: *Essential Otolaryngology*, p. 718)**

470. (A) Untreated, furunculosis can cause serious complications such as cavernous sinus thrombosis. **(Ref: *Essential Otolaryngology*, p. 719)**

471. (E) Swearinger (1965) determined that the nasoethmoidal complex has a maximum tolerable impact force before fracture of 35 to 80 g. These forces are relatively small when compared to those required for other fractures of the facial skeleton. (**Ref:** *Otolaryngology—Head and Neck Surgery,* **p. 737**)

472. (**D**) Fluorescein injection and then observing the appropriately placed pledgets (middle meatus, cribiform plate, sphenoethmoid recess) can usually localize the site of a CSF leak. (**Ref:** *Essential Otolaryngology,* **p. 722**)

473. (**E**) Posterior inferior bleeding is usually from the sphenopalatine vessels, while superior bleeding usually is from the anterior and posterior ethmoid vessels. (**Ref:** *Essential Otolaryngology,* **pp. 722–723**)

474. (**C**) Angiography before arterial ligation is recommended if there is evidence of flow from the contralateral carotid system, history of transient ischemic episode or CVA, or physical evidence of carotid artery disease or vascular compromise of the globe (amaurosis fugax). (**Ref:** *Otolaryngology—Head and Neck Surgery,* **pp. 132–134**)

475. (**D**) Approximately 50% of children with choanal atresia have other defects such as Treacher Collins syndrome, branchial arch anomalies, and cardiac or gut abnormalities. (**Ref:** *Otolaryngology—Head and Neck Surgery,* **pp. 711–712**)

476. (**B**) This nipple acts as an oropharyngeal airway through which the baby can breathe. Feeding can also be a major problem as children tend to swallow air while feeding. (**Ref:** *Otolaryngology—Head and Neck Surgery,* **p. 712**)

477. (**D**) With vasomotor rhinitis, there is usually an increase in acetylcholine in nasal mucosa characterized by increased parasympathetic tone. (**Ref:** *Essential Otolaryngology,* **p. 724**)

478. (**E**) Wegener granulomatosis is associated with necrotizing granulomas with vasculitis involving the respiratory tract and kidney (necrotizing glomerulonephritis). (**Ref:** *Essential Otolaryngology,* **p. 725**)

479. (**D**) This is an extremely rare tumor but it is very radiosensitive. (**Ref:** *Essential Otolaryngology,* **p. 728**)

480. (E) Parosmia is a condition in which there is a perverted sense of smell. This may occur as a result of injury to the uncus of the temporal lobe. **(Ref: *Essential Otolaryngology*, p. 730)**

481. (A) Inverted papillomas are usually unilateral, with a preponderance in men. They may resemble nasal polyps but are less translucent. **(Ref: *Essential Otolaryngology*, p. 731)**

482. (E) The middle turbinate is an osseous shelf approximately 3.5 to 4.0 cm in length and is sometimes pneumatized with an ethmoid cell (4 to 12%). **(Ref: *Essential Otolaryngology*, pp. 734–735)**

483. (A) Mucormycosis is very common in the debilitated patient but does not show this pattern on x-ray. **(Ref: *Essential Otolaryngology*, p. 673)**

484. (D) Paranasal sinus malignant tumors are rare. After squamous cell carcinoma, the most common malignant tumor of the paranasal sinus is adenoid cystic carcinoma, undifferentiated transitional cell carcinoma, adenocarcinoma, and malignant melanoma. **(Ref: *Essential Otolaryngology*, pp. 744–745)**

485. (C) In frontal sinusitis, when the infection spreads to become osteomyelitis of the frontal bone, a subperiosteal abscess develops over the anterior surface. This is called a Pott puffy tumor. **(Ref: *Otolaryngology—Head and Neck Surgery*, p. 936)**

36

The Larynx

DIRECTIONS (Questions 486 through 500): Each of the numbered items or incomplete statements in this section is followed by answers or completions of the statement. Select the ONE lettered answer or completion that is BEST in each case.

486. Some of the extrinsic muscles of the larynx depress the larynx as a whole and these include the sternohyoid, thyrohyoid, and
  A. omohyoid
  B. geniohyoid
  C. digastrics
  D. mylohyoid
  E. stylohyoid

487. The muscle that is the main abductor of the vocal cord is the
  A. lateral cricoarytenoid
  B. cricothyroid
  C. interarytenoid
  D. posterior cricoarytenoid
  E. thyroarytenoid

488. The external branch of the superior laryngeal nerve (SLN) supplies motor function to the following muscle
   A. interarytenoid
   B. cricothyroid
   C. posterior cricoarytenoid
   D. thyroarytenoid
   E. lateral cricoarytenoid

489. A 4-year-old child presents to the emergency department with sudden onset of progressive dyspnea and is leaning forward. The first step in management is
   A. to start an intravenous
   B. to examine the oral cavity and pharynx with a tongue depressor
   C. not to stimulate the child, order a portable lateral neck x-ray, and prepare the operating room
   D. to administer racemic epinephrine
   E. to obtain blood work

490. A 55-year-old male presents with a slowly progressive dyspnea and hoarseness. Indirect laryngoscopy reveals a smooth, round lesion covered with normal mucosa on the internal aspect of the posterior plate of the cricoid cartilage. The most likely diagnosis is
   A. granular cell myoblastoma
   B. papilloma
   C. chondroma
   D. neurofibroma
   E. chemodectoma

491. Intubation granuloma can be seen after endotracheal intubation. On indirect laryngoscopy, the lesion is seen in the following anatomic position on the vocal cords
   A. anterior ⅓
   B. junction of anterior ⅓, posterior ⅔
   C. midvocal cords
   D. posterior ⅓
   E. vocal process of the arytenoid

492. A 60-year-old male has a vocal cord biopsy because of a hyperplastic and keratinized lesion in the posterior commissure. Histology shows acanthosis, parakeratosis, keratosis, and hyperkeratotic papilloma with no dyskeratosis. The diagnosis is
   A. sarcoidosis
   B. pseudoepithelial hyperplasia
   C. papilloma
   D. pachyderma laryngis
   E. diphtheritic laryngitis

493. With long-term endotracheal intubation, the incidence of subglottic stenosis is
   A. < 1%
   B. 1 to 3%
   C. 5 to 10%
   D. 10 to 15%
   E. > 15%

494. A 3-month-old female infant presents with mild inspiratory stridor and a history of repeated croup-like episodes. Direct laryngoscopy reveals a pink to blue compressible subglottic tumor. The next step in management is to
   A. biopsy the mass
   B. perform bronchoscopy past the lesion to assess the lower trachea
   C. stop the procedure at this point and discuss with the parents about later YAG or CO_2 laser excision
   D. excise the lesion
   E. perform an emergency tracheotomy

495. A 6-month-old female infant presents with a history of a weak, wailing cry, rounded facies, and hypotonia. The next step in management is
   A. chromosomal testing
   B. CAT scan of the larynx
   C. tracheotomy
   D. direct laryngoscopy
   E. observation for 3 to 6 months

496. Paralysis of the laryngeal muscles results from the peripheral motor nerve in the following percentage of cases
   A. 10%
   B. 30%
   C. 50%
   D. 90%
   E. 70%

497. The clinical test that is used to help diagnose superior laryngeal nerve paralysis is the
   A. Guttman test
   B. Lillie–Crowe test
   C. DiSant' Agnese test
   D. Mollaret–Debre test
   E. Sulkowitch test

498. The CO_2 laser emits a beam of light of
   A. 6.1 μm
   B. 8.5 μm
   C. 2.3 μm
   D. 0.5 μm
   E. 10.6 μm

499. At the time of surgery, a 6-year-old male has a bleeding subglottic hemangioma. The most appropriate laser to use is the
   A. argon
   B. YAG
   C. CO_2
   D. KTP-532
   E. KTP-400

500. One of the biggest advantages of the argon laser over the CO_2 laser is that
   A. the beam has less scatter
   B. the beam can be transmitted through fiberoptic cables
   C. ordinary glasses can protect your eyes from damage
   D. the absorption is not dependent on the color of the tissue
   E. it is less costly to operate

The Larynx

ANSWERS AND DISCUSSION

486. **(A)** The geniohyoid, digastrics, mylohyoid, and stylohyoid are elevators of the larynx. (**Ref:** *Essential Otolaryngology,* **p. 762**)

487. **(D)** The posterior cricoarytenoid muscle passes from the posterior surface of the cricoid lamina to the muscular process of the arytenoid cartilage. It also causes lateral rotation of the arytenoids. (**Ref:** *Essential Otolaryngology,* **pp. 762–763**)

488. **(B)** The recurrent (inferior) laryngeal nerve (RLN) supplies motor innervation to all the intrinsic laryngeal muscles of the same side, except for the cricothyroid, and to the interarytenoid muscle on both sides. (**Ref:** *Otolaryngology—Head and Neck Surgery,* **p. 1701**)

489. **(C)** The primary diagnosis to rule out is epiglottitis. Any stimulation of the child could cause complete airway obstruction. (**Ref:** *Essential Otolaryngology,* **p. 770**)

490. **(C)** In most cases, the mass is situated posteriorly and laterally. Most pathologists feel that chondromas and the low grade chondrosarcomas are so similar that the histologic distinction between them has little practical experience. (**Ref:** *Otolaryngology—Head and Neck Surgery,* **p. 1921**)

491. (E) Intubation granuloma occurs when mucosal healing is incomplete. Perichondritis persists and granulation tissue remains in a localized area. **(Ref: *Otolaryngology—Head and Neck Surgery*, p. 1886)**

492. (D) Pachyderma laryngis is not a premalignant condition and treatment is nonspecific. **(Ref: *Essential Otolaryngology*, p. 783)**

493. (B) This problem occurs most frequently in children because the subglottis is the narrowest part of their upper airway. Other etiologic factors are external trauma, post-tracheotomy, burns, neoplasm, irradiation, infection, or congenital. **(Ref: *Essential Otolaryngology*, pp. 787–788)**

494. (C) This may be a subglottic capillary hemangioma and biopsy could lead to a major bleed. **(Ref: *Essential Otolaryngology*, pp. 789–790)**

495. (A) This most likely represents cri-du-chat syndrome. The larynx has the same appearance as that seen in laryngeal chrondromalacia. **(Ref: *Essential Otolaryngology*, pp. 790–791)**

496. (D) The vagus nerve arises from the ambiguous nucleus in the midbrain. Paralysis of the vocal cords can be described as median, paramedian, intermediate, and extreme abduction (lateral). **(Ref: *Essential Otolaryngology*, p. 794)**

497. (A) The Guttman sign is associated with superior laryngeal nerve paralysis. In the normal individual, pressure over the thyroid cartilage causes an increased voice pitch, whereas anterior pressure causes a decrease. In SLN paralysis, the reverse is true. **(Ref: *Essential Otolaryngology*, pp. 800–801)**

498. (E) Due to its specific wavelength and beam coherence capability, the CO_2 laser vaporizes tissue precisely with minimal surrounding thermal damage and is therefore used frequently for microlaryngeal surgery. **(Ref: *Essential Otolaryngology*, p. 812)**

499. (B) The YAG laser has an invisible beam of light at 1.06 μm. It is an excellent photocoagulator. It has a 20 to 40% scatter and penetrates deeply. **(Ref: *Essential Otolaryngology*, p. 813)**

500. (B) One of the disadvantages of the argon laser is that it operates on a 220-volt energizer and an open cooling system, requiring both a voltage adapter and an exterior plumbing and cooling system. **(Ref: *Essential Otolaryngology*, pp. 812–813)**

37

Sleep Apnea

DIRECTIONS (Questions 501 through 510): Each of the numbered items or incomplete statements in this section is followed by answers or completions of the statement. Select the ONE lettered answer or completion that is BEST in each case.

501. Apnea is defined as the cessation of airflow at the nostrils and mouth for at least
   A. 3 seconds
   B. 5 seconds
   C. 10 seconds
   D. 20 seconds
   E. 30 seconds

502. You send a patient for a sleep study. If his sleep study is abnormal, he would have an apnea index of
   A. 1 or greater
   B. 2 or greater
   C. 3 or greater
   D. 4 or greater
   E. 5 or greater

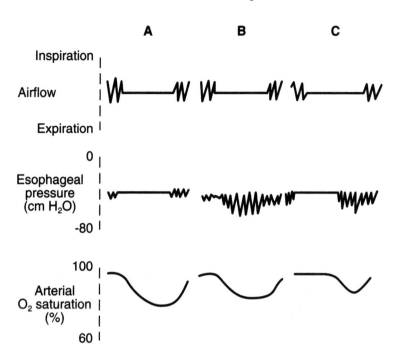

503. The above pattern is consistent with obstructive sleep apnea
    A. A
    B. B
    C. C
    D. A or B
    E. B or C

504. The incidence of sleep apnea is greater in males than females by a ratio of
    A. 4:1
    B. 6:1
    C. 8:1
    D. 20:1
    E. 30:1

505. Sleep apnea has been associated with high serum levels of
    A. urobilinogen
    B. progesterone
    C. testosterone
    D. thyroxine
    E. adrenaline

506. You send a patient for a sleep latency test. The results are normal. The normal range is
    A. 5 to 10 minutes
    B. 10 to 15 minutes
    C. 15 to 20 minutes
    D. 20 to 25 minutes
    E. 25 to 30 minutes

507. Nasal continuous positive airway pressure (CPAP) may be the treatment of choice for many sleep apnea patients and the effective pressure ranges are from
    A. 1 to 5 cm H_2O
    B. 5 to 20 cm H_2O
    C. 20 to 50 cm H_2O
    D. 50 to 75 cm H_2O
    E. 75 to 100 cm H_2O

508. Narcolepsy can be confirmed by the presence of
    A. REM-onset sleep during a daytime sleep study
    B. a prolonged NREM sleep pattern
    C. a ratio of REM/NREM sleep of 1:1
    D. continuous REM sleep at night
    E. high progesterone levels on blood testing

509. Oxygen desaturation is usually more severe with
    A. mixed apnea
    B. central apnea
    C. obstructive sleep apnea
    D. narcolepsy
    E. snoring

510. A 45-year-old male who has moderate sleep apnea and severe snoring is going to have a septoplasty and UPPP. He wants to know what percentage of patients will have a significant improvement in snoring. You say

A. 30%

B. 30 to 40%

C. 40 to 50%

D. 70 to 80%

E. > 95%

Sleep Apnea

ANSWERS AND DISCUSSION

501. **(C)** Apnea is defined as the cessation of airflow at the nostrils and mouth for at least 10 seconds. Obstructive apnea is a cessation of airflow in the presence of continued inspiratory effort. Central apnea is the absence of both airflow and inspiratory effort. Mixed apnea is a combination of both of the above. **(Ref:** *Otolaryngology—Head and Neck Surgery,* **p. 1392)**

502. **(E)** An apnea index is the average number of apneas per hour of sleep. The respiratory disturbance index is the average number of apneas plus hypopneas per hour of sleep. If either of these indexes is below 5, this is considered normal. Clinically symptomatic patients usually have an apnea index greater than 30. **(Ref:** *Essential Otolaryngology,* **p. 826)**

503. **(B)** Obstructive apnea is characterized by absence of airflow and presence of continued respiratory effort. Note the corresponding drop in arterial oxygen saturation with all types of apnea. **(Ref:** *Otolaryngology—Head and Neck Surgery,* **p. 1393)**

504. **(C)** Men are eight times more likely to develop obstructive sleep apnea than are women. Men also tend to have more severe sleep apnea. **(Ref:** *Essential Otolaryngology,* **p. 827)**

505. (C) High levels of testosterone have been associated with sleep apnea. In contrast, progesterone may contribute to a low frequency of disordered breathing during sleep in premenopausal women. **(Ref:** *Otolaryngology—Head and Neck Surgery,* **p. 1396)**

506. (B) The mean sleep latency measures the amount of time required for a patient to fall asleep. The mean sleep latency in normal persons is 10 to 15 minutes. **(Ref:** *Otolaryngology—Head and Neck Surgery,* **p. 1399)**

507. (B) CPAP effective pressure ranges from 5.0 to 20.0 cm H_2O. Because the pressure needed to eliminate apneas and hypopneas varies in patients, they should be introduced to nasal CPAP in the laboratory so that the proper pressure can be determined. **(Ref:** *Essential Otolaryngology,* **p. 830)**

508. (A) Narcolepsy is a sleep disorder characterized by episodes of sudden onset of sleep of short duration. It is confirmed by the presence of REM-onset sleep during a daytime sleep study. **(Ref:** *Otolaryngology—Head and Neck Surgery,* **pp. 1400– 1401)**

509. (C) With severe obstructive apnea, there is usually more significant oxygen desaturation. **(Ref:** *Essential Otolaryngology,* **p. 835)**

510. (D) Approximately 75 to 80% of patients will have a significant improvement in snoring. **(Ref:** *Otolaryngology—Head and Neck Surgery,* **p. 1405)**

38

Facial and Airway Trauma

DIRECTIONS (Questions 511 through 525): Each of the numbered items or incomplete statements in this section is followed by answers or completions of the statement. Select the ONE lettered answer or completion that is BEST in each case.

511. A 30-year-old male had a traumatic puncture hole in the infraauricular area with complete facial nerve paralysis on that side. Electrical stimulation is possible for the distal nerve. It is best to
    A. explore the wound within 3 days and repair the nerve
    B. wait for at least 10 days until initial wound healing is achieved
    C. wait 20 days until the nerve can maximally synthesize protein
    D. wait 3 months, then repair
    E. consider electrical testing of the nerve daily for 1 week

512. A 20-year-old female is diagnosed as having a mandible fracture by the radiologist. Without looking at the x-rays, the most likely area of the mandible fracture is the
    A. coronoid
    B. angle
    C. condyle

    D. ramus

    E. body

513. The four muscles that are important elevators of the mandible are the temporalis, masseter, lateral ptergoid, and

    A. digastric

    B. genioglossus

    C. geniohyoid

    D. mylohyoid

    E. medial pterygoid

514. You suspect a patient has a condyle fracture. Probably the best x-ray to obtain for this is a (an)

    A. Towne view

    B. posterior anterior (PA) view

    C. occlusal view

    D. oblique

    E. anteroposterior (AP) view

515. You are asked to see a 55-year-old alcoholic who had an undiagnosed comminuted fracture that is now 4 days postinjury and is infected. The best treatment would be

    A. the use of arch bars

    B. internal fixation with interosseous wiring

    C. internal fixation with miniplates

    D. internal fixation with direct compression plates

    E. external (pin) fixation

516. A 6-year-old boy falls from his bike and presents to the emergency room with subcutaneous emphysema on the left side of his cheek. He most probably has a fracture of the

    A. nasal process of the frontal bone

    B. lamina papyracea

    C. ethmoid bulla

    D. crista galli

    E. frontal process of the maxilla

517. A 35-year-old female presents to the emergency room with typical signs of a malar fracture. If you only had one x-ray to order, this one would give you the most information.
  A. lateral
  B. submental vertex
  C. waters
  D. Caldwell
  E. modified towns

518. The intraoral approach to zygomatic fractures is termed the
  A. Gillies approach
  B. Keen approach
  C. transantral approach
  D. Adam approach
  E. Ludwig approach

519. The floor of the orbit is composed primarily of the following bone
  A. frontal
  B. lacrimal
  C. palatine
  D. zygomatic
  E. maxillary

520. With orbital fractures, the technique of applying local anesthetic and grasping the sclera at the insertion of the inferior rectus tendon and finding limited rotation of the globe is termed
  A. forced duction test
  B. Guttman test
  C. Schirmer test
  D. DiSant'Agnese test
  E. Sulkowitch test

521. A 25-year-old male after a motor vehicle accident has x-rays taken that show a pyramidal fracture from the pterygoid plate through the infraorbital rim and the nasal–frontal suture. He has a classification called a
  A. Le Fort I fracture
  B. severe nasoethmoid fracture
  C. Le Fort II fracture
  D. nasal fracture
  E. Le Fort III fracture

522. The most accepted treatment for a frontal sinus fracture that is linear and minimally displaced is
A. exploration and elevation
B. exploration and frontal sinus obliteration
C. exploration and packing the frontal sinus
D. observation
E. external fixation

523. A 30-year-old female had a previous frontal fracture that was moderately comminuted and was treated with observation. She presents 6 months later to a physician with chronic headaches. The most likely diagnosis is
A. mucocele
B. temporal arteritis
C. CSF leak
D. migraines secondary to head trauma
E. psychosomatic disease

524. A 25-year-old male presents to emergency after a motor vehicle accident with hoarseness, cervical subcutaneous emphysema, and loss of palpable laryngeal prominences. The next step in management is
A. direct laryngoscopy
B. Gastrografin swallow
C. external manipulation of the neck
D. prepare for tracheotomy, as this may be necessary
E. insert a standard endotracheal tube

525. The second most frequently fractured facial bone is the
A. zygoma
B. nasal bone
C. maxilla
D. frontal bone
E. mandible

Facial and Airway Trauma

ANSWERS AND DISCUSSION

511. (A) When immediate complete paralysis is a result of laceration or penetrating trauma, exploration should be within 3 days from the time of injury. The distal nerve can still be stimulated at this point. If it does not stimulate, repair is best achieved on the 20th day, as the nerve can maximally synthesize protein at this point. **(Ref:** *Essential Otolaryngology,* **p. 840)**

512. (C) Condyle fractures occur 36% of the time, while body is approximately 21%, angle is 20%, parasymphyseal is 14%, ramus is 3%, alveolar is 3%, and symphyseal is 1%. **(Ref:** *Essential Otolaryngology,* **p. 842)**

513. (E) Depressor–retractor muscles of the mandible are the digastric, geniohyoid, genioglossus, and the mylohyoid. **(Ref:** *Otolaryngology—Head and Neck Surgery,* **p. 381)**

514. (A) A CT scan is the best modality to assess any fractures in the head and neck area. **(Ref:** *Essential Otolaryngology,* **p. 843)**

515. (E) External (Pin) fixation is indicated where there are multiple comminuted fractures, infected fractures, and where MMF is contraindicated because of alcoholism or psychiatric illness. Its disadvantage is that it is very cumbersome. **(Ref:** *Essential Otolaryngology,* **p. 844)**

516. (B) Severe injuries to the lamina papyracea and nasoethmoidal complex can be very challenging. There may be damage to the lacrimal apparatus, medial canthal ligaments, superior orbital muscle, and nasofrontal duct obliteration. **(Ref: *Otolaryngology—Head and Neck Surgery*, pp. 391–392)**

517. (C) Submental vertex view is best for arch fractures, but of course the best modality for accessing any fractures is the CT scan. **(Ref: *Essential Otolaryngology*, p. 847)**

518. (B) The Gillies approach is the most common reduction technique to use for zygomatic fractures. This procedure should be delayed until the edema following trauma settles, as this technique relies heavily on palpation and external visualization of the position of the zygoma. **(Ref: *Otolaryngology—Head and Neck Surgery*, p. 387)**

519. (E) The orbital plate of the maxilla forms a large aspect of the medial floor of the orbit. This will usually fracture on the floor of orbit fractures. Fortunately, the orbital floor projection of the zygoma usually remains intact. **(Ref: *Otolaryngology—Head and Neck Surgery*, p. 391)**

520. (A) This positive forced duction test indicates an orbital floor fracture with muscle entrapment as there is limited rotation. **(Ref: *Essential Otolaryngology*, p. 849)**

521. (C) A Le Fort III fracture is when there is cranial dysjunction from the pterygoid plate through the frontozygomatic suture, orbit, and nasal frontal suture. In a Le Fort I fracture, there is a transverse fracture from the pterygoid plate to the nasal pyramid. **(Ref: *Essential Otolaryngology*, p. 851)**

522. (D) It is important to rule out any future cosmetic deformity and also if there are any fragments of bone obstructing the nasofrontal duct or CSF leak. **(Ref: *Otolaryngology—Head and Neck Surgery*, p. 382)**

523. (A) A mucocele can develop as a result of nasofrontal duct obstruction or entrapment of mucosa in the posterior table fracture.

This is why it is so important to fully assess frontal sinus fractures early with CT scanning and try to prevent later sequelae. (**Ref:** *Essential Otolaryngology,* **p. 852**)

524. (**D**)   One should be totally prepared to maintain or establish an airway as any manipulation on physical examination may compromise this. Indirect laryngoscopy, CT scanning, Gastrografin swallow may all be helpful after one is prepared to do an emergency tracheotomy. (**Ref:** *Essential Otolaryngology,* **p. 854**)

525. (**E**)   The nose is the most frequently fractured facial bone. (**Ref:** *Essential Otolaryngology,* **p. 845**)

39

Pediatric Otolaryngology

DIRECTIONS (Questions 526 through 540): Each of the numbered items or incomplete statements in this section is followed by answers or completions of the statement. Select the ONE lettered answer or completion that is BEST in each case.

---

526. The cranium has reached 90% of the adult size by age
   A. 3 years
   B. 4 years
   C. 5 years
   D. 6 years
   E. 7 years

527. The eustachian tube is approximately this length at birth
   A. 10 mm
   B. 17 mm
   C. 22 mm
   D. 30 mm
   E. 39 mm

528. The percentage of children who have had at least one episode of otitis media by age 3 is
A. 25%
B. 40%
C. 50%
D. 70%
E. 95%

529. In children with multiple sclerosis, vertigo is the presenting symptom the following percentage of the time
A. 5%
B. 10%
C. 20%
D. 40%
E. 60%

530. A 5-year-old male patient has a rhabdomyosarcoma of the pharynx resected with positive regional lymph nodes. The pathology report shows regional disease with involved nodes grossly resected and evidence of microscopic residual disease. This stage would be
A. group I b
B. group II b
C. group II c
D. group III
E. group IV

531. A 6-year-old boy is brought to your office 5 days after sustaining a severe laceration to his face. He also suffered an immediate facial paralysis. On maximum stimulation test of the distal segment, one would expect the response to be
A. 0
B. 1.0 to 2.0 ma
C. 2.0 to 3.0 ma
D. 3.0 to 4.0 ma
E. > 4.0 ma

532. The maxillary sinuses appear at approximately
 A. birth
 B. 1 year
 C. 2 years
 D. 3 years
 E. 4 years

533. You are asked to see a newborn who has choanal atresia. The incidence of ear abnormalities associated with this is approximately
 A. 10%
 B. 30%
 C. 40%
 D. 60%
 E. 90%

534. The incidence of choanal atresia is approximately
 A. 1 in 1000 births
 B. 1 in 3000 births
 C. 1 in 5000 births
 D. 1 in 10,000 births
 E. 1 in 20,000 births

535. The following percentage of facial fractures occur in children of age 0 to 5 years
 A. 1%
 B. 5%
 C. 10%
 D. 15%
 E. 20%

536. The incidence of malignant melanoma in giant congenital nevi is approximately
 A. 1%
 B. 5%
 C. 12%
 D. 20%
 E. 50%

537. A 6-year-old patient has a group A beta-hemolytic streptococci. His mother asks what the incidence is of developing rheumatic fever if the child is not treated. You tell her the incidence is
   A. 1%
   B. 3%
   C. 10%
   D. 15%
   E. 20%

538. A 5-year-old female has mumps. Her mother is worried because she is very drowsy and has difficulty arousing her. The incidence of meningoencephalitis with mumps is
   A. 1%
   B. 2.5%
   C. 10%
   D. 15%
   E. 20%

539. A 5-year-old male swallowed an unknown agent and died 12 hours later. The autopsy showed there was liquefaction necrosis of the esophageal wall. A possible agent would be
   A. hydrochloric acid
   B. sulfuric acid
   C. nitric acid
   D. sodium hydroxide
   E. bleach

540. A 4-year-old male aspirated a peanut. You would expect to find it in the following area on bronchoscopy
   A. right bronchus
   B. left bronchus
   C. hypopharynx
   D. trachea
   E. larynx

Pediatric Otolaryngology

ANSWERS AND DISCUSSION

526. (C) The cranium has reached 90% of its adult size by age 5. **(Ref:** *Essential Otolaryngology,* **p. 857)**

527. (B) The eustachian tube at birth is approximately 17 mm, which is about one half the adult length. The nasopharyngeal opening is at the level of the hard palate at birth and inferior turbinate by age 6. This is important with regard to eustachian tube dysfunction. **(Ref:** *Essential Otolaryngology,* **p. 858)**

528. (D) Approximately 71% of children have had one or more episodes of otitis media by age 3. **(Ref:** *Pediatric Otolaryngology,* **p. 324)**

529. (C) Approximately 20% of children with multiple sclerosis will present with vertigo. **(Ref:** *Essential Otolaryngology,* **p. 862)**

530. (C) Group II c is regional disease with involved nodes grossly resected but with evidence of microscopic residual disease. Group III is incomplete resection or biopsy with gross residual disease and group IV is metastatic disease present at onset. **(Ref:** *Pediatric Otolaryngology,* **p. 1348)**

531. (A) It has been shown that a completely sectioned nerve may continue to conduct distal to the section for as long as 48 to 72 hours after the injury. For this reason, the MST has limited value until 48 to 72 hours after the onset of the paralysis. **(Ref: *Pediatric Otolaryngology*, p. 258)**

532. (A) The maxillary sinuses are present at birth. **(Ref: *Essential Otolaryngology*, p. 864)**

533. (E) Approximately 88% of children who are born with choanal atresia will have ear abnormalities (deafness, pinna anomalies, etc.). **(Ref: *Essential Otolaryngology*, p. 864)**

534. (C) The incidence of choanal atresia occurs in 1 in 5000 births. Unilateral atresia is twice as common as bilateral disease and bony atresia is more common than membranous. **(Ref: *Essential Otolaryngology*, p. 864)**

535. (A) A child's facial skeleton is very elastic and only 1% of all fractures occur in children of age 0 to 5 years. **(Ref: *Essential Otolaryngology*, p. 867)**

536. (C) These giant congenital nevi have to be watched very carefully. Growth and change in pigmentation are danger signs and the incidence of malignant melanoma is 72%. **(Ref: *Essential Otolaryngology*, p. 870)**

537. (B) The incidence of acquiring rheumatic fever after untreated group A beta-hemolytic streptococci is approximately 3%. **(Ref: *Essential Otolaryngology*, p. 872)**

538. (B) The incidence of meningoencephalitis is 25%. **(Ref: *Essential Otolaryngology*, p. 873)**

539. (D) Acids cause coagulation necrosis and alkalis cause liquefaction necrosis. Therefore, the only alkali on the list is sodium hydroxide. **(Ref: *Pediatric Otolaryngology*, p. 998)**

540. (A) The most common site of an aspirated foreign body lodging is the right bronchus (48%). Approximately 29% will lodge in the left bronchus. **(Ref: *Essential Otolaryngology*, p. 879)**

40

Pediatric Airway and Laryngeal Problems

DIRECTIONS (Questions 541 through 550): Each of the numbered items or incomplete statements in this section is followed by answers or completions of the statement. Select the ONE lettered answer or completion that is BEST in each case.

---

541. A 4-month-old child is seen in consultation for stridor that has persisted for 2 months. According to the mother, the child improves if placed in the prone position. The most probable diagnosis is

   A. laryngocele
   B. laryngomalacia
   C. subglottic stenosis
   D. vocal cord paralysis
   E. foreign body aspiration

542. A 6-year-old male sustained a clothesline injury to the neck while riding his bicycle. He presents to the emergency room 1 hour later with a small amount of hemoptysis and hoarseness. Your treatment is
    A. IV steroids and send home
    B. racemic epinephrine and send home
    C. direct laryngoscopy and observation for at least 12 hours
    D. observation for 3 hours and send home if no deterioration of symptoms
    E. IV fluids, possible intubation

543. An 18-month-old female presents with mild stridor. On laryngoscopy, you note a lesion that clinically is a small to moderate sized hemangioma. Correct treatment would be
    A. laser therapy
    B. radiotherapy
    C. chemotherapy
    D. steroid injection
    E. close observation

544. The incidence of subglottic stenosis in neonates after prolonged intubation is
    A. < 8%
    B. 8 to 20%
    C. 20 to 30%
    D. 30 to 40%
    E. 40 to 50%

545. The following is not true of a juvenile nasopharyngeal angiofibroma
    A. patients range from age 7 to 21 years
    B. the incidence in females is greater than in males
    C. most common vascular mass in the nasopharynx
    D. carotid arteriography is virtually diagnostic
    E. it is slowly progressive

546. The criteria for performing an anterior cricoid split procedure for treatment of acquired subglottic stenosis is true in all of the following except
    A. greater than 1500 gm weight
    B. no assisted ventilation for 10 days before evaluation

C. supplemental O_2 requirement less than 30%
D. extubation failure on at least two occasions secondary to laryngeal pathologic conditions
E. no congestive heart failure for 1 month prior to evaluation

547. A child with subglottic stenosis has approximately a 70 to 90% laryngeal lumen obstruction. He/she is a grade
A. I
B. II
C. III
D. IV
E. V

548. A 3-year-old male aspirated a foreign body. An appropriate diameter scope to use would be
A. 2.0 mm
B. 3.0 mm
C. 4.0 mm
D. 5.0 mm
E. 6.0 mm

549. HPV-11 is identified in a lesion of the larynx in an 8-year-old child. The most probable diagnosis is
A. chondroma
B. subglottic hemangioma
C. leiomyoma
D. recurrent respiratory papillomatosis
E. neurofibromatosis

550. The major risk in treatment of subglottic hemangioma with CO_2 laser treatment is
A. bleeding
B. subglottic scarring or stenosis
C. infection
D. edema formation
E. tracheal perforation

Pediatric Airway and Laryngeal Problems

ANSWERS AND DISCUSSION

541. (B)   Laryngomalacia accounts for 60% of all laryngeal problems in infants. The child is usually worse in the supine position and improves in the prone position. (**Ref:** *Essential Otolaryngology,* **p. 892)**

542. (C)   With blunt trauma to the neck, one has to be concerned that edema will get worse over 6 to 12 hours. Also, hemoptysis indicates there may be serious internal damage to the larynx or esophagus. (**Ref:** *Pediatric Otolaryngology,* **pp. 1180–1181)**

543. (E)   If there is only mild stridor and no other airway problems, then close observation is appropriate. Subglottic hemangiomas grow in size until the child is about age 2 years, then involute spontaneously. (**Ref:** *Essential Otolaryngology,* **p. 893)**

544. (A)   Only 1 to 8% of neonates develop subglottic stenosis. It has been shown that neonates re-epithelialize subglotticly even though the endotracheal tube is kept in place. (**Ref:** *Pediatric Otolaryngology,* **p. 1194)**

545. (B) When a girl is diagnosed with juvenile nasopharyngeal angiofibroma, then the physician should question the diagnosis and possibly perform chromosome studies on the patient. **(Ref: *Essential Otolaryngology*, p. 901)**

546. (A) A neonate must be at least 1500 g in order to perform an anterior cricoid split procedure. **(Ref: *Pediatric Otolaryngology*, p. 1197)**

547. (B) A grade II is a 70 to 90% lumen obstruction, while a grade I is less than 70%. A grade III is greater than 90%, while a grade IV is complete obstruction. **(Ref: *Pediatric Otolaryngology*, p. 1199)**

548. (C) For 3- or 4-year-old children, an appropriate scope would be 4.0 mm. **(Ref: *Pediatric Otolaryngology*, p. 1211)**

549. (D) HPV-11 and HPV-6 have been identified as the viral subtypes in laryngeal papillomatosis. **(Ref: *Pediatric Otolaryngology*, p. 1215)**

550. (B) The major concern with laser treatment of subglottic hemangioma is the development of subglottic scarring. **(Ref: *Pediatric Otolaryngology*, p. 1219)**

41

Facial Plastic Surgery

DIRECTIONS (Questions 551 through 570): Each of the numbered items or incomplete statements in this section is followed by answers or completions of the statement. Select the ONE lettered answer or completion that is BEST in each case.

551. The deepest point in the nasofrontal angle is called the
- **A.** sallion
- **B.** nasion
- **C.** radix
- **D.** sill
- **E.** rhinion

552. All of the following are nasal tip support mechanisms except
- **A.** size, shape, and resilience of medial and lateral crura
- **B.** attachment of medial crural footplate to the caudal border of the quadrangular cartilage
- **C.** attachment of the caudal order of the upper lateral cartilage to the cephalic border of the lower lateral cartilage
- **D.** attachment of septum to ethmoid plate
- **E.** cartilaginous septal dorsum

553. The ideal columella–labial angle in a female is
- **A.** 100 to 110°
- **B.** 95 to 100°

C. 90 to 95°
D. 110 to 115°
E. 115 to 120°

554. The Frankfort horizontal plane extends from the infraorbital rim to the
   A. inferior border of the external auditory canal
   B. superior border of the external auditory canal
   C. midaspect of the external auditory canal
   D. pinna of the ear
   E. tragus of the ear

555. In external septorhinoplasty, the columella incision should be
   A. at the level of the inferior attachment of medial crura
   B. above the level of the inferior attachment of medial crura
   C. below the level of the inferior attachment of medial crura
   D. anywhere on the columella
   E. at the base of the columella

556. A marginal incision is located at
   A. the inferior border of the lower lateral cartilage
   B. the superior border of the lower lateral cartilage
   C. the inferior border of the upper lateral cartilage
   D. the inferior border of medial crura
   E. the level of interior septal angle

557. The single most important factor in increasing tip support is
   A. not using an intracartilaginous incision
   B. using a medial crura strut
   C. using a hemitransfixion incision
   D. using an intradomal suture
   E. not dividing the lower lateral crura

558. A useful test to determine the presence of an abnormality of the vestibular portion of the nasal valve is the
   A. Guttman test
   B. Schirmer test
   C. Lillie–Crowe test
   D. Bunnell test
   E. Cottle test

559. The tragus and crus helicus of the ear are derived from the following branchial arch
   A. first
   B. second
   C. third
   D. fourth
   E. fifth

560. During otoplasty, removal of postauricular skin or mastoid soft tissue may result in
   A. a telephone ear deformity
   B. a hematoma
   C. recurrence of defect
   D. a helial deformity
   E. a Mustardé defect

561. A 55-year-old female about to undergo lower lid blepharoplasty has a positive pinch test. One should
   A. consider taking more lower lid skin than previously indicated
   B. consider removing more fat
   C. consider a lid-shortening procedure at the same time
   D. consider a skin flap only
   E. consider a transconjunctival approach only

562. A 45-year-old female patient has mild ectropion laterally 2 days after surgery. You should
   A. consider steroid injection
   B. reassure the patient this will resolve
   C. consider a skin graft
   D. remove some sutures
   E. use steroid ointment

563. During upper lid blepharoplasty, the surgeon inadvertently picked up orbital septum with an eyelid skin closure suture. This may result in
   A. ectropion
   B. lagophthalmos
   C. ptosis
   D. epiphora
   E. conjunctival edema

564. During upper lid blepharoplasty, the most common injury that can cause diplopia is an injury to the
   A. supratrochlear muscle
   B. superior oblique muscle
   C. lateral rectus muscle
   D. medial rectus muscle
   E. orbital septum

565. A face lift patient with anterior banding of the platysma muscle that is either in repose or accentuated by voluntary contraction is considered a
   A. Class I
   B. Class II
   C. Class III
   D. Class IV
   E. Class V

566. The average incidence of hematoma formation after rhytidectomy is
   A. < 1%
   B. 3%
   C. 7%
   D. 20%
   E. 25%

567. In suction lipectomy, one requires at least the following level of negative pressure to achieve smooth continuous fat extraction
   A. 0.40 atmospheres of negative pressure
   B. 0.50 atmospheres of negative pressure
   C. 0.60 atmospheres of negative pressure
   D. 0.70 atmospheres of negative pressure
   E. 0.80 atmospheres of negative pressure

568. The increase in length of the central limb is dependent on the size of the angles of a Z-plasty. An angle of 60° gives the following increase in length
   A. 40%
   B. 55%
   C. 73%
   D. 80%
   E. 92%

569. Tunable dye lasers emit energy between
   - **A.** 540 and 545 nm
   - **B.** 560 and 565 nm
   - **C.** 577 and 585 nm
   - **D.** 588 and 600 nm
   - **E.** 601 and 608 nm

570. A port wine stain, in which the vessels no longer can be distinguished and there is no normal tissue between the ectatic blood vessels, is considered a grade
   - **A.** I
   - **B.** II
   - **C.** III
   - **D.** IV
   - **E.** V

Facial Plastic Surgery

ANSWERS AND DISCUSSION

551. (A) The sellion is the deepest point in the nasofrontal angle. The nasion is the anatomic midpoint of the nasofrontal suture and is higher than the sellion. **(Ref: *Aesthetic Facial Surgery*, p. 38)**

552. (D) All are correct except the attachment of the septum to the ethmoid plate. **(Ref: *Essential Otolaryngology*, p. 912)**

553. (A) The ideal columella–labial angle is 100 to 110° in females and 95 to 100° in men. **(Ref: *Aesthetic Facial Surgery*, p. 37)**

554. (B) The Frankfort horizontal plane is important in photography for proper facial analysis. **(Ref: *Aesthetic Facial Surgery*, p. 48)**

555. (B) If the incision is placed at or below the level of the inferior attachment of medial crura, it can cause notching or retraction. **(Ref: *Aesthetic Facial Surgery*, p. 103)**

556. (A) A marginal or rim incision is located at the inferior border of the lower lateral cartilage. **(Ref: *Aesthetic Facial Surgery*, p. 73)**

557. (B) To stabilize or increase the projection of a nose, a strut is the single most important factor. (**Ref:** *Aesthetic Facial Surgery,* **pp. 88–89**)

558. (E) The Cottle test is done while the patient breathes quietly. The cheek is drawn laterally away from the midline, opening the nasal valve angle. The patient is asked if this maneuver improves airflow through the test side. If this occurs, it is a positive Cottle sign and indicates the abnormality of the vestibular portion of the nasal valve that contributes to the symptomatic nasal obstruction. (**Ref:** *Aesthetic Facial Surgery,* **p. 177**)

559. (A) Only the tragus and crus helicus are derived from the first branchial arch. Eighty-five percent of the auricle is derived from the second arch. (**Ref:** *Aesthetic Facial Surgery,* **p. 708**)

560. (A) A telephone ear deformity after otoplasty may be the result of excessive removal of skin in the middle third segment of the ear, excessive resection of mastoid soft tissues, or excessive tightening of concha mastoid sutures. (**Ref:** *Aesthetic Facial Surgery,* **p. 732**)

561. (C) A pinch test is done to evaluate tonicity of the lower lid. If this is very lax, a lid-shortening procedure should be done to avoid potential ectropion. (**Ref:** *Essential Otolaryngology,* **pp. 917–918**)

562. (B) After surgery, it is not unusual to have mild ectropion that is transient and is related to edema. (**Ref:** *Essential Otolaryngology,* **pp. 922–923**)

563. (B) Lagophthalmos can result from the orbital septum being picked up inadvertently. It will usually resolve spontaneously. (**Ref:** *Essential Otolaryngology,* **p. 922**)

564. (B) If superior oblique muscle injury occurs and is unrecognized, it may be necessary to explore the superior oblique muscle. (**Ref:** *Essential Otolaryngology,* **p. 923**)

565. (D)   A class IV patient has anterior banding of the platysma muscle, while class III has excessive fat in the submandibular and/or submental areas. **(Ref: *Essential Otolaryngology*, p. 924)**

566. (C)   The average incidence of hematoma after rhytidectomy is 7%. **(Ref: *Essential Otolaryngology*, p. 927)**

567. (D)   One requires at least 20 inches of mercury or 0.70 atmospheres of negative pressure to achieve smooth, continuous fat extraction. **(Ref: *Aesthetic Facial Surgery*, p. 693)**

568. (C)   An angle of 45° on a Z-plasty gives an increase in length of 50%, while an angle of 60° gives a 73% increase in length. **(Ref: *Essential Otolaryngology*, p. 935)**

569. (C)   The tunable dye laser emits energy between 577 and 585 nm. Oxyhemoglobin in port wine stains has maximum absorption at 418, 542, and 577 nm. **(Ref: *Essential Otolaryngology*, p. 937)**

570. (D)   In a port wine stain, grade IV is vessels that are no longer distinguished and there is no normal tissue between the ectatic blood vessels. These vessels are raised and vary from light to dark purple. **(Ref: *Essential Otolaryngology*, p. 938)**

42

Head and Neck Reconstructive Surgery

DIRECTIONS (Questions 571 through 580): Each of the numbered items or incomplete statements in this section is followed by answers or completions of the statement. Select the ONE lettered answer or completion that is BEST in each case.

---

571. The blood supply for the deltopectoral flap is from the
    A. external carotid artery
    B. internal carotid artery
    C. internal mammary artery
    D. brachiocephalic artery
    E. subclavian artery

572. In raising the deltopectoral flap, one should be careful not to damage the following vein
    A. cephalic
    B. internal mammary
    C. subclavian
    D. internal jugular
    E. brachiocephalic

573. The major disadvantage of the deltopectoral flap is that
    A. it cannot be used in a patient who has had radiation
    B. it has a poor blood supply
    C. a second operation is usually required
    D. it is not commonly used for floor of mouth defects
    E. it is a small flap

574. The strongest and most dependable blood supply of a regional flap is the
    A. deltopectoral flap
    B. rhomboid flap
    C. pectoralis musculocutaneous flap
    D. forehead flap
    E. nape of neck flap

575. The blood supply of the pectoralis musculocutaneous flap is from the
    A. thoracoacromial artery
    B. internal mammary artery
    C. subclavian artery
    D. internal carotid artery
    E. intercostal arteries

576. The major disadvantage of the pectoralis musculocutaneous flap is that it
    A. has a poor blood supply
    B. requires a two-stage operation
    C. is a very bulky flap
    D. requires more technical expertise than a free flap
    E. is not a free flap

577. The main blood supply of the trapezius musculocutaneous flap is the
    A. suprascapular artery
    B. transverse cervical artery
    C. dorsal scapular artery
    D. occipital artery
    E. subclavian artery

578. The musculocutaneous flap with the most tenuous blood supply is the
  A. pectoralis
  B. latissimus dorsi
  C. deltopectoral
  D. trapezius
  E. sternocleidomastoid

579. With free revascularized tissue transfer grafts, the following percentage of grafts are unsuccessful in the first 24 to 72 hours
  A. < 5%
  B. 5 to 15%
  C. 15 to 25%
  D. 25 to 30%
  E. > 30%

580. In order to try to avoid a "no-reflow" phenomenon, the ideal enteric flap ischemia time should optimally be less than
  A. 15 minutes
  B. 2 hours
  C. 2.5 hours
  D. 3 hours
  E. 4 hours

Head and Neck Reconstructive Surgery

ANSWERS AND DISCUSSION

571. (C) The deltopectoral flap is based on three or four perforating branches of the internal mammary artery. When designed in a length/width ratio of more than 2.5:1, it may be used without delay. (**Ref:** *Otolaryngology—Head and Neck Surgery,* **pp. 1294–1296**)

572. (A) The flap is elevated deep to the fascia in a lateral to a medial direction. Care should be taken not to damage the cephalic vein. (**Ref:** *Essential Otolaryngology,* **pp. 946–947**)

573. (C) To achieve the desired length necessary to close most oral cavity or pharyngeal defects, a delay procedure is necessary. (**Ref:** *Essential Otolaryngology,* **p. 946**)

574. (D) The forehead flap has its blood supply from the superficial temporal and occipital arteries of the external carotid system. It can be used on a nondelay basis for a variety of reconstructive techniques. The flap has a limited use because it is quite aesthetically unacceptable. (**Ref:** *Otolaryngology—Head and Neck Surgery,* **p. 462**)

575. (A) The pectoralis musculocutaneous flap is the most commonly used of the musculocutaneous flaps because it is dependable and versatile. (**Ref:** *Essential Otolaryngology,* **p. 951**)

576. (C) The major advantage of this flap is that it allows transfer of a distinct amount of skin into a deficit, which permits suturing of the entire circumference in a one-stage reconstruction. (**Ref:** *Otolaryngology—Head and Neck Surgery,* **p. 1492**)

577. (B) The blood supply to this flap is the transverse cervical artery. (**Ref:** *Essential Otolaryngology,* **p. 953**)

578. (E) The sternocleidomastoid flap is actually not a true musculocutaneous flap because there is a layer of muscle interposed between the skin island and the major muscle providing the blood supply for the skin island. (**Ref:** *Essential Otolaryngology,* **p. 956**)

579. (B) Revascularized free flaps circumvent many of the limitations imposed by regional flaps. The large number of free-flap donor sites has expanded the reconstructive possibilities for a large skin, soft tissue, and composite defects of the head and neck. (**Ref:** *Essential Otolaryngology,* **p. 960**)

580. (B) Complete regeneration of the endothelium across a microvascular anastomosis takes 2 weeks. During this interval, collagen fibers are exposed to elements of the blood and place the vessel at risk for thrombosis. (**Ref:** *Essential Otolaryngology,* **p. 961**)

43

Anesthesia for Head and Neck Surgery

DIRECTIONS (Questions 581 through 590): Each of the numbered items or incomplete statements in this section is followed by answers or completions of the statement. Select the ONE lettered answer or completion that is BEST in each case.

581. According to the American Society of Anesthesiologists, a patient with insulin-dependent diabetes would be considered an ASA class
    A. I
    B. II
    C. III
    D. IV
    E. V

582. A 40-year-old female patient is allergic to PABA. When administering local anesthesia, one should not use
    A. mepivacaine
    B. cocaine
    C. tetracaine
    D. lidocaine
    E. bupivacaine

583. The maximum single dose of xylocaine with epinephrine that can safely be given as a maximum single dose is
  A. 100 mg
  B. 200 mg
  C. 300 mg
  D. 400 mg
  E. 500 mg

584. This agent causes disassociative anesthesia, which results from the selective disruption of association pathways of the brain before a somataesthetic sensory blockade is produced. This agent is
  A. diazepam
  B. midazolam hydrochloride
  C. fentanyl
  D. ketamine hydrochloride
  E. methohexital sodium

585. The incidence of allergic reaction to local anesthesia is approximately
  A. 2%
  B. 5%
  C. 7%
  D. 10%
  E. 12%

586. The maximum recommended dose of cocaine is
  A. 1 mg/kg
  B. 2 to 3 mg/kg
  C. 5 mg/kg
  D. 7 to 8 mg/kg
  E. 10 mg/kg

587. A severe reaction that can occur as a result of bupivacaine (Marcaine) overdose is
  A. cardiovascular collapse
  B. liver toxicity
  C. CNS depression
  D. hypertension
  E. aplastic anemia

588. The onset of action for tetracaine hydrochloride (Pontocaine) is
   A. 1 to 2 minutes
   B. 2 to 4 minutes
   C. 6 to 12 minutes
   D. 12 to 20 minutes
   E. > 20 minutes

589. Amide-type drugs are metabolized in the
   A. GI tract
   B. liver
   C. kidney
   D. plasma
   E. spleen

590. The duration of the analgesic effect of cocaine on nasal mucosa is
   A. 10 minutes
   B. 20 minutes
   C. 30 minutes
   D. 45 minutes
   E. 60 minutes

Anesthesia for Head and Neck Surgery

ANSWERS AND DISCUSSION

581. (C)   An ASA class III is a patient with severe disease that limits activity but is not incapacitating (marked hypertension, insulin-dependent diabetes, etc.). (**Ref:** *Aesthetic Facial Surgery,* **p. 503**)

582. (B)   Cocaine is an ester linkage local anesthetic and ester compounds are also derivatives of para-aminobenzoic acid (PABA). Allergic reactions to ester compounds are more common in patients with allergies to PABA. (**Ref:** *Aesthetic Facial Surgery,* **p. 505**)

583. (E)   ASU single dose 500 mg of xylocaine with adrenaline can be given, while only 300 mg (30 m/s of 1%) without epinephrine can be given. (**Ref:** *Aesthetic Facial Surgery,* **p. 506**)

584. (D)   Ketamine hydrochloride has a unique analgesic and anesthetic effect that causes the patient to be neither asleep nor anesthetized but instead subdued, entranced, and disassociated from the surroundings. (**Ref:** *Aesthetic Facial Surgery,* **p. 507**)

585. (B)   True allergic reactions to local anesthetics are approximately 2%. (**Ref:** *Essential Otolaryngology,* **p. 972**)

586. (B) Cocaine is an extremely potent topical anesthetic agent and the maximum recommended dose is 2 to 3 mg/kg. **(Ref:** *Essential Otolaryngology,* **p. 975)**

587. (A) Bupivacaine (Marcaine) toxicity can result in intractable seizures and cardiovascular collapse. **(Ref:** *Essential Otolaryngology,* **p. 976)**

588. (C) The onset of action of tetracaine hydrochloride (Pontocaine) is 6 to 12 minutes and prolonged duration of action is 1.5 to 2 hours. **(Ref:** *Essential Otolaryngology,* **p. 975)**

589. (B) Amide-type drugs are metabolized by the liver, while ester-type drugs are hydrolyzed by cholinesterases in the liver and plasma. **(Ref:** *Essential Otolaryngology,* **p. 970)**

590. (D) Cocaine effect is immediate and the duration is approximately 45 minutes. **(Ref:** *Essential Otolaryngology,* **p. 975)**

44

Head and Neck Radiology

DIRECTIONS (Questions 591 through 600): Each of the numbered items or incomplete statements in this section is followed by answers or completions of the statement. Select the ONE lettered answer or completion that is BEST in each case.

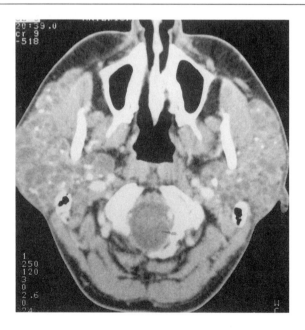

591. The above MRI scan is consistent with
   A. bilateral Warthin syndrome
   B. Sjögren syndrome
   C. Heffer disease
   D. parotid abscess
   E. normal hypertrophied parotid glands

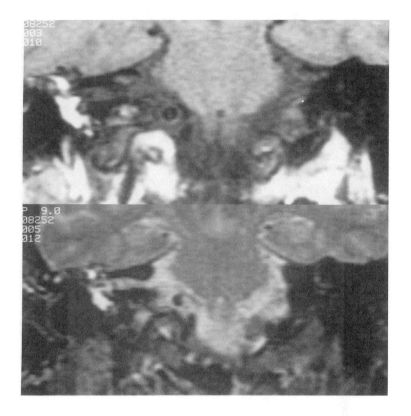

592. The above MRI scan (T_1 image) of the middle ear is consistent with
   A. cholesterol granuloma
   B. cholesteatoma
   C. squamous cell carcinoma
   D. ossicular discontinuity
   E. serous otitis media

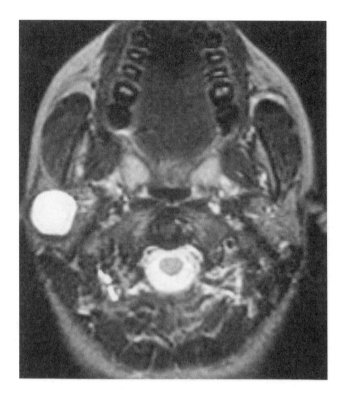

593. The above MRI scan is consistent with a diagnosis of
   A. Warthin tumor of the parotid gland
   B. hemangioma of the parotid gland
   C. type I branchial cleft cyst of the parotid gland
   D. abscess of the parotid gland
   E. Sjögren syndrome

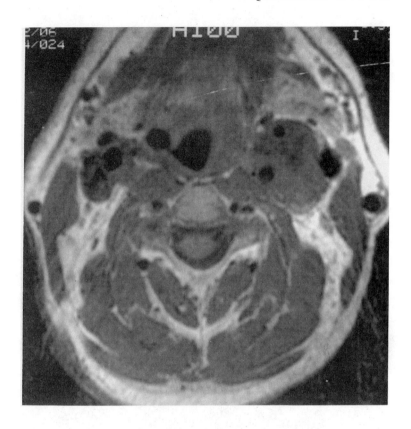

594. The above MRI scan of the neck is consistent with the diagnosis of
   A. squamous cell carcinoma of the neck
   B. lymphadenopathy
   C. parotid tumors
   D. vagal paragangliomas
   E. branchial cleft cyst

595. Normal salivary glands will expel contrast material from the gland within a certain time. This is usually within
   A. 2 minutes
   B. 5 minutes
   C. 20 minutes
   D. 60 minutes
   E. 6 hours

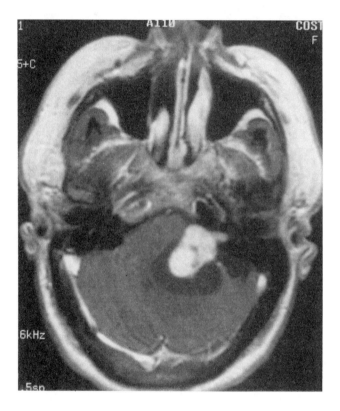

596. The above MRI scan is consistent with the diagnosis of a (an)
   A. cerebellar tumor
   B. cholesterol granuloma
   C. cholesteatoma
   D. brain abscess
   E. acoustic neuroma

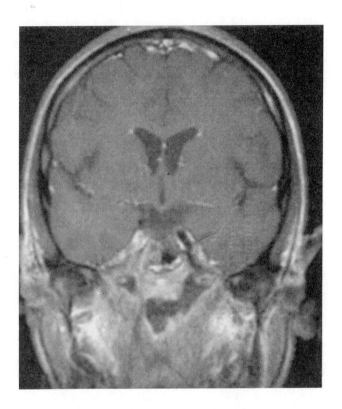

597. The above patient has AIDS. The most likely diagnosis is
   A. extensive mucormycosis of the sinuses
   B. nasal polyps
   C. antrochoanal polyps
   D. carcinoma of the nasopharynx
   E. acute bacterial sinusitis

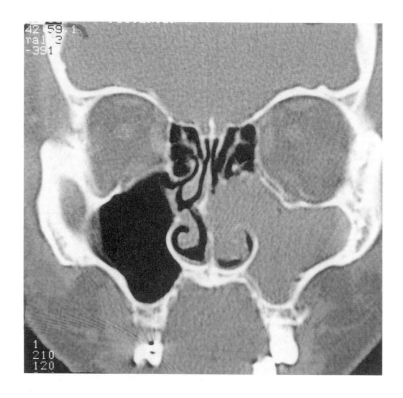

598. The above MRI scan is consistent with
 A. nasal polyps
 B. inverting papillomas
 C. acute maxillary sinusitis
 D. oral antral polyp
 E. mucocele

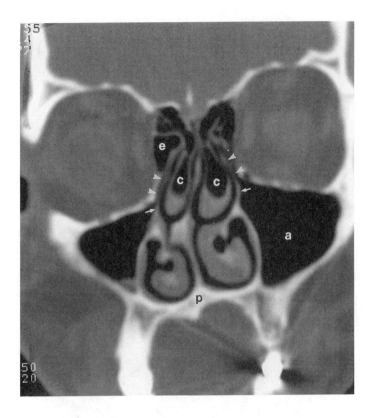

599. The letter "c" in the above MRI scan indicates
   A. bilateral conchal bullosa
   B. bilateral nasal polyps
   C. bilateral mucoceles
   D. bilateral osteomeatal complex narrowing
   E. normal anatomy

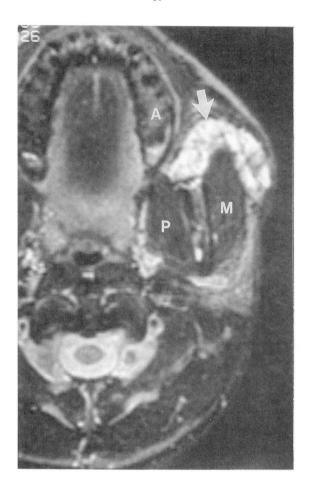

600. The arrow in this MRI scan (T_1) of the cheek is pointing toward a
  A. hemangioma of the cheek
  B. parotid tumor
  C. facial abscess
  D. acute maxillary sinusitis
  E. trigeminal neuroma

I wish to thank Helmuth W. Gahbauer, MD, Attending Radiologist, Hospital of Saint Raphael, New Haven, Connecticut, for his assistance in completing this chapter.

Head and Neck Radiology

ANSWERS AND DISCUSSION

591. (B) Sjögren's syndrome is the second most common connective tissue disease after rheumatoid arthritis. Fifty percent of patients have salivary gland enlargement. The enlargement is more commonly diffuse rather than modular. (**Ref:** *Otolaryngology—Head and Neck Surgery,* **p. 1037**)

592. (A) Cholesterol granuloma on MRI scan lights up on T_1 and T_2 images. A similar pattern would be seen with blood in the middle ear space. (**Ref:** *Otolaryngology—Head and Neck Surgery,* **pp. 2736–2737**)

593. (C) This MRI is consistent with a type I branchial cleft cyst of the parotid gland. (**Ref:** *Essential Otolaryngology,* **p. 1043**)

594. (D) Approximately 3% of all paragangliomas originate from the vagus nerve. In this case they are bilateral. (**Ref:** *Otolaryngology—Head and Neck Surgery,* **pp. 1590–1597**)

595. (B) The normal salivary gland expels the contrast within 5 minutes. (**Ref:** *Essential Otolaryngology,* **p. 1019**)

596. (E) This is an example of a large acoustic neuroma. (**Ref:** *Essential Otolaryngology,* **p. 1038**)

597. (A) This is an example of extensive mucormycosis with invasion of the skull base. (**Ref:** *Otolaryngology—Head and Neck Surgery*, **pp. 931–933)**

598. (B) This is an example of inverted papilloma. The incidence of frank malignant change approximates 10%. (**Ref:** *Otolaryngology—Head and Neck Surgery*, **p. 948)**

599. (A) This indicates bilateral conchal bullosa. These may have to be crushed or removed in order to perform endoscopic sinus surgery. (**Ref:** *Otolaryngology—Head and Neck Surgery*, **pp. 630–631)**

600. (A) This is a facial hemangioma extending around the anterior aspect of the masseter muscle. (**Ref:** *Otolaryngology—Head and Neck Surgery*, **pp. 325–326)**

45

Pharmacology and Therapeutics

DIRECTIONS (Questions 601 through 610): Each of the numbered items or incomplete statements in this section is followed by answers or completions of the statement. Select the ONE lettered answer or completion that is BEST in each case.

---

601. A patient of yours was administered ketoconazole (Nizoral). He was also on terfenadine. He then developed an abnormality on his ECG. One would expect to see
  - **A.** prolonged PR interval
  - **B.** inverted T waves
  - **C.** shortened PR interval
  - **D.** prolonged QT interval
  - **E.** suppressed QRS wave

602. One of the major side effects of the H_2-receptor antagonists is
  - **A.** reduction of hepatic blood flow thus reducing metabolism of various drugs
  - **B.** tachycardia
  - **C.** drowsiness
  - **D.** blurred vision
  - **E.** acute glaucoma

287

603. The following drug has its mechanism of action as a competitive inhibition of acetylcholine at muscarinic sites
   A. azatadine
   B. meclizine
   C. promethazine
   D. scopolamine
   E. ketoconazole

604. In the case of a severe allergic reaction, the time of onset of IV corticosteroids is
   A. immediately
   B. 10 to 20 minutes
   C. 20 to 40 minutes
   D. 40 to 60 minutes
   E. 60 to 120 minutes

605. Salicylates can cause reversible hearing loss and tinnitus. Generally, the serum level must be above
   A. 5 mg/dL
   B. 10 mg/dL
   C. 15 mg/dL
   D. 20 mg/dL
   E. 30 mg/dL

606. The average dose of streptomycin sulfate in the treatment of intractable bilateral Ménière disease is
   A. 250 mg per day
   B. 500 mg per day
   C. 2 g per day
   D. 4 g per day
   E. 6 g per day

607. A 20-year-old female had a tonsillectomy and was given medication postoperatively. Later, her mother phones to tell you she has become lethargic and is making involuntary, dyskinetic movements. This is probably related to the following medication
   A. Demerol
   B. codeine

    C. prochlorperazine (Compazine)
    D. acetaminophen
    E. penicillin

608. One of the following medications has a mechanism of action of blocking reuptake of catecholamines at sympathetic nerve terminals
    A. Otrivin
    B. lidocaine
    C. prochlorperazine
    D. quinine
    E. cocaine

609. The following medication has been implicated in the cause of gingival hyperplasia in about 25% of chronically treated patients
    A. furosemide
    B. nitrogen mustard
    C. diphenylhydantoin (Dilantin)
    D. quinine
    E. scopolamine (Hyoscine)

610. Desmopressin (DDAVP) has been found to increase temporarily the concentration of factor
    A. V
    B. VI
    C. VII
    D. VIII
    E. IX

Pharmacology and Therapeutics

ANSWERS AND DISCUSSION

601. **(D)** Terfenadine and ketoconazole or erythromycin-based products have been implicated in ECG abnormalities, including QT internal prolongation and toursades de pointes (polymorphic ventricular tachycardia). (**Ref:** *Essential Otolaryngology,* p. 1068)

602. **(A)** H_2-receptor antagonists are associated with mental status changes, antiandrogenic effects, but especially a reduction of hepatic blood flow, thus reducing the metabolism of various drugs, which may accumulate in toxic concentrations. (**Ref:** *Essential Otolaryngology,* p. 1068)

603. **(D)** Drugs in this class are anticholinergics and scopolamine is the most effective drug for motion sickness, with fewer side effects than the others in its class. (**Ref:** *Essential Otolaryngology,* pp. 1068–1069)

604. **(E)** Corticosteroids should not replace epinephrine in the treatment of severe allergic hypersensitivity, as they are not effective until at least 60 to 120 minutes after administration. (**Ref:** *Essential Otolaryngology,* p. 1071)

605. (D) To produce ototoxicity with salicylates, 6 to 8 grams per day must be taken, resulting in a serum level of 20 mg/dL or greater. **(Ref: *Essential Otolaryngology*, p. 1073)**

606. (C) The usual dose of streptomycin sulfate in the treatment of intractable bilateral Ménière disease is 2 g per day until no caloric response is elicited. **(Ref: *Essential Otolaryngology*, p. 1073)**

607. (C) Prochlorperazine (Compazine) can cause tardive dyskinesia, a syndrome consisting of potentially irreversible, involuntary, dyskinetic movements. The treatment is to stop the medication, administer Benadryl, and observe. **(Ref: *Essential Otolaryngology*, p. 1070)**

608. (E) Cocaine has a potent effect via blocking reuptake of catecholamines at sympathetic nerve terminals in addition to a role as local anesthetic. **(Ref: *Essential Otolaryngology*, p. 1070)**

609. (C) Gingival hyperplasia occurs in about 25% of chronically treated patients taking diphenylhydantoin (Dilantin) and is the most common adverse reaction in children and adolescents. **(Ref: *Essential Otolaryngology*, pp. 1075–1076)**

610. (C) Desmopressin (DDAVP) has been found to increase temporarily the concentration of factor VII: C antihemophilic factor and Von Willebrand factor in blood. **(Ref: *Essential Otolaryngology*, pp. 1079–1080)**

46

Miscellaneous Information

DIRECTIONS (Questions 611 through 630): Each of the numbered items or incomplete statements in this section is followed by answers or completions of the statement. Select the ONE lettered answer or completion that is BEST in each case.

611. The contents of the superior orbital fissure include the superior ophthalmic vein, the inferior ophthalmic vein branch, V_1 nerve branches, and the following nerves
    A. II, IV, V_2, and VI
    B. II and IV
    C. II, IV, V_3, and VI
    D. II, IV, and VI
    E. II, III, IV, and VI

612. The V_2 cranial nerve exits the skull via the
    A. foramen lacerum
    B. foramen ovale
    C. foramen rotundum
    D. foramen spinosum
    E. hypoglossal canal

613. The esophageal dehiscence between the cricopharyngeus and the circular fibers of the esophagus is called by the following name
  A. Killian
  B. Killian–Jamieson
  C. Lamier–Hackman
  D. Winkler–Jamieson
  E. Winkler

614. The most common complication of cholesteatoma is
  A. serous or suppurative labyrinthitis
  B. semicircular canal erosion/fistula and disequilibrium
  C. facial nerve paralysis
  D. Bezold abscess
  E. brain abscess

615. Numbness of the postauricular area associated with compression of the facial nerve by an acoustic neuroma is called
  A. Hitselberger sign
  B. Leopold sign
  C. Sewell sign
  D. Ramsay sign
  E. Guttman sign

616. The percentage of patients who have a family history of otosclerosis is
  A. 25%
  B. 50%
  C. 75%
  D. 60%
  E. 100%

617. The following test is used to diagnose gustatory sweating after parotidectomy
  A. Guttman
  B. Guyon
  C. Minor
  D. Goodwin
  E. Brooke

618. A 70-year-old male has been diagnosed on biopsy of having a metastatic malignant tumor of the temporal bone. The most probable site of the primary tumor is the
  A. prostate
  B. liver
  C. colon
  D. testes
  E. parotid

619. A 6-year-old girl is having a T&A. Suddenly, her temperature increases, her pulse increases, and the patient becomes rigid. One should discontinue anesthetic agents, administer 100% oxygen, cool the patient, and give intravenous
  A. digoxin
  B. Xylocaine
  C. Diamox
  D. dantrolene
  E. calcium chloride

620. An 18-month-old male presented with fever, proptosis, hepatomegaly, multiple bony lesions, and exfoliative dermatitis. The child died in 4 months. The most probable diagnosis was
  A. eosinophilic granuloma
  B. acute mylogenous leukemia
  C. Hand–Schüller–Christian disease
  D. acute lymphosarcoma
  E. Letterer–Siwe disease

621. A 66-year-old female presents with oral bullae. Biopsy shows autoantibodies, acantholysis, and a positive Nikolsky sign. The diagnosis is
  A. pemphigoid
  B. squamous cell carcinoma
  C. pemphigus
  D. granular cell myoblastoma
  E. lichen planus

622. The following percentage of basilar skull fractures have CSF otorrhea
- **A.** < 2%
- **B.** 10%
- **C.** 6%
- **D.** 20%
- **E.** 30%

623. The incidence of metastases of squamous cell carcinoma of the lower lip is
- **A.** 1 to 3%
- **B.** > 30%
- **C.** 6 to 8%
- **D.** 10 to 12%
- **E.** 20 to 30%

624. The most common soft tissue malignancy in the head and neck in children is
- **A.** granular cell myoblastoma
- **B.** histiocytosis X
- **C.** squamous cell carcinoma
- **D.** rhabdomyosarcoma
- **E.** craniopharyngioma

625. A 50-year-old male presents with left upper cervical lymphadenopathy. Needle aspiration reveals squamous cell carcinoma and workup is negative for a primary. His 5-year survival with treatment is
- **A.** 10%
- **B.** 50%
- **C.** 30%
- **D.** 70%
- **E.** 90%

626. The most frequent virus to be associated with the common cold is
- **A.** enterovirus
- **B.** adenovirus
- **C.** influenza virus
- **D.** parainfluenza virus
- **E.** rhinovirus

627. A 70-year-old male has a loss of sense of taste, vocal cord paralysis, palate paralysis, and limited movement of his shoulder and tongue. He has the following syndrome
A. Vernet
B. Schmidt
C. Villaret
D. Collet–Sicard
E. Avellis

628. A 17-year-old female presents with a diffuse painless swelling of the left cheek. X-rays reveal a ground glass, multilocular appearance with diffuse margins. The most likely diagnosis is
A. fibrous dysplasia
B. ossifying fibroma
C. Wegener granulomatosis
D. Hand–Schüller–Christian disease
E. eosinophilic granuloma

629. The incidence of malignant melanoma is 7/100,000 and of these the following percentage is found in the head and neck region
A. 5%
B. 10%
C. 30%
D. 20%
E. 50%

630. Malignant melanoma classification of 3.60 mm: non-BANS according to the modified Breslow staging has a 5-year survival rate of
A. 20%
B. 50%
C. 30%
D. 70%
E. 90%

Miscellaneous Information

ANSWERS AND DISCUSSION

611. (D) The inferior orbital fissure contains V_2 branches (zygomatic nerves and sphenopalatine branch) and the inferior ophthalmic vein. (**Ref:** *Essential Otolaryngology,* **p. 1143)**

612. (C) The V_1 comes through the superior orbital fissure and the V_3 comes through the foramen ovale. (**Ref:** *Essential Otolaryngology,* **p. 1143)**

613. (B) The Killian dehiscence is between the cricopharyngeus and the thyropharyngeus muscles and the Lamier–Hackman dehiscence is between the circular and longitudinal fibers of the esophagus. (**Ref:** *Essential Otolaryngology,* **p. 1147)**

614. (B) After semicircular canal erosion and fistula, the most common complications of cholesteatoma are extradural or perisinus abscess; serous or suppurative labyrinthitis; facial nerve paralysis; meningitis; epidural, subdural or parenchymal brain abscess; and recurrent cholesteatoma. (**Ref:** *Essential Otolaryngology,* **p. 1086)**

615. (A) This is a very rare sign of an acoustic neuroma. (**Ref:** *Essential Otolaryngology,* **p. 1090)**

616. **(B)** With otosclerosis, it is most common in Caucasians and women are twice as often afflicted as are men. Pregnancy often coincides with the onset of otosclerosis or an increase in lesion activity. **(Ref: *Essential Otolaryngology*, p. 685)**

617. **(C)** This is a starch–iodine test. Iodine is painted on the patient's face and is allowed to dry. Starch is dusted onto the skin. Then, a sialogogue is used. If Frey syndrome is present, black spots will appear in the starch. **(Ref: *Essential Otolaryngology*, p. 1093)**

618. **(A)** Bony metastases to the temporal bone can also originate from the breast, kidney, lung, stomach, larynx, and colon. **(Ref: *Essential Otolaryngology*, p. 1094)**

619. **(D)** Malignant hyperthermia is caused by the release of calcium in large amounts from the sarcoplasmic reticulum, usually associated with the use of depolarizing anesthetic agents. **(Ref: *Essential Otolaryngology*, p. 1099)**

620. **(E)** Letterer–Siwe disease is a rapidly progressive disease that is almost always fatal. Hand–Schüller–Christian disease has a 30% mortality. **(Ref: *Essential Otolaryngology*, p. 1101)**

621. **(C)** Pemphigus has oral manifestations in 66% of cases. Steroids are the method of treatment. **(Ref: *Essential Otolaryngology*, p. 1107)**

622. **(C)** Approximately 90% of basilar skull fractures heal spontaneously. **(Ref: *Essential Otolaryngology*, p. 1109)**

623. **(C)** Basal cell carcinoma is most often associated with upper lip lesion. Squamous cell carcinoma of the upper lip often will metastasize early. **(Ref: *Essential Otolaryngology*, p. 1110)**

624. **(D)** Rhabdomyosarcomas most often present before age 10. Orbital tumors are unique in that they tend toward locally aggressive behavior but rarely metastasize. The converse is true of other sites. **(Ref: *Essential Otolaryngology*, p. 1111)**

625. (C)   The prognosis is worse if the primary lesion is discovered. **(Ref: *Essential Otolaryngology*, p. 1110)**

626. (E)   Other viruses associated with the common cold include coronaviruses, parainfluenza virus, respiratory syncytial virus, adenovirus, enterovirus, influenza virus, and reovirus. **(Ref: *Essential Otolaryngology*, p. 1138)**

627. (D)   The etiology of this syndrome is usually a meningioma or other lesion involving the nerves in the posterior cranial fossa. **(Ref: *Essential Otolaryngology*, p. 225)**

628. (A)   The appearance of bone in fibrous dysplasia has been described as "ground glass." The bone proliferation of fibrous dysplagia should not be confused with an osteoma, in which the margin of the dense bone mass is usually much more sharply defined. **(Ref: *Otolaryngology—Head and Neck Surgery*, pp. 921–923)**

629. (D)   There are two staging criteria for malignant melanoma, which are directly related to prognosis. One is the Clark staging and the other is the modified Breslow staging. **(Ref: *Essential Otolaryngology*, p. 1137)**

630. (D)   Modified Breslow staging of 0.85 mm and 0.85 to 1.70 mm: non-BANS have a 5-year survival rate of 99%. BANS and 1.70 to 3.60 mm: non-BANS have a 5-year survival rate of 75%. BANS has a 0% 5-year survival rate. **(Ref: *Essential Otolaryngology*, p. 1137)**

New Edition!

Essential Otolaryngology Head & Neck Surgery

A Board Preparation and Concise Review

Sixth Edition

K. J. Lee, MD, FACS

Whether you're a resident, fellow, practicing ENT, or surgeon, *Essential Otolaryngology, 6/e* provides a concise yet substantial review of the field. This new edition features over 1200 pages of vital information and is highly illustrated with line drawings, photos, x-rays, tables, and graphs. Written in expanded outline format, chapters are divided by subject, and are contributed by over fifty specialists.

1995, 1296 pp., 233 illus., P, ISBN 0-8385-2214-9, A2214-3

Available at your local health science bookstore or call 1-800-423-1359 (in CT 838-4400).

Appleton & Lange • 25 Van Zant Street • P. O. Box 5630 • Norwalk, CT • 06856